An Educational Challenge: Meeting the Needs of Students with Brain Injury

By
Dana S. DeBoskey, Ph.D.

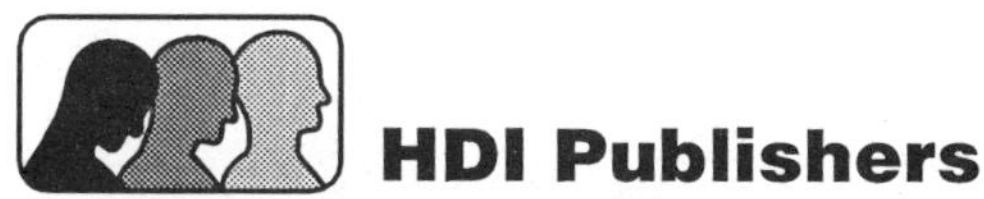

Printed in the United States of America on acid free paper. ∞

Library of Congress Cataloging-in-Publication Data

DeBoskey, Dana S.

An educational challenge : meeting the needs of students with brain injury / Dana S. DeBoskey.

p. cm.

Includes bibliographical references.

ISBN 1-882855-37-X (alk. paper). - - ISBN 1-882855-37-X (alk. paper)

1. Brain-damaged children--Education--United States. 2. Brain-damaged children--Rehabilitation--United States. I. Title.

[DNLM: WS 340 D287e 1995]

LC4596.D43 1996

371.91 ' 6--dc20

DNLM/DLC

95-50380

CIP

AN EDUCATIONAL CHALLENGE: MEETING THE NEEDS OF STUDENTS WITH BRAIN INJURY

This manual was developed and produced
for use in teacher and family education
by DeBoskey and Associates, Tampa, Florida.
Other volumes by DeBoskey and Associates published
by HDI include:

Coming Home: A Discharge Manual for Families of the Brain Injured

Working After Brain Injury: What Can I Do?

Pain: Making Life Liveable

The author would like to gratefully acknowledge
the contributions of the following persons:

Gary M. Pace, Ph.D.
Deborah C. Schultz, M.S.
Allen W. Freeman, M.Ed.
Charlotte A. Hooker, M.A.
JoEllen W. Preston, M.A.
Thomas W. Oleson, M.S.
Joan M. Dye, M.S.

For a complete catalog of
HDI's brain injury resources contact:

HDI Publishers
P.O. Box 131401
Houston, TX 77219
Toll Free (800) 321-7037
Fax (713) 956-2288

DEDICATION

This manual is dedicated to all the teachers who are struggling to understand and address the special needs of students who are brain injured, and to the parents who desire an appropriate education for their injured child.

TABLE OF CONTENTS

PREFACE

There is much disagreement among educators, and particularly educational administrators, as to how the educational needs of children with brain injury can best be met. The focus of this thinking is often guided by factors and contingencies that are not understood by those outside the educational arena. Or, if understood, there is not a sense of acceptance of the limitations set forth. It is difficult to explain to parents why their child must be placed within an "educational category" that does not truly represent the disability.

Essentially, there are two schools of thought concerning the needs of a child who is brain injured. On the one hand, there are those who believe these needs can best be met through the currently existing programs, or at least a combination of programs. This would necessitate that all special education teachers, as well as regular classroom teachers, receive training in this area of specialty. It also necessitates that there be some degree of flexibility in entrance criteria to specific programs. This plan, however, is fraught with problems in choosing the best placement.

The other school of thought would like to see specialized classes and a recognized category of teachers established to handle students who are brain injured. This would have to start at the federal level so that specific full-time teaching units could be set aside. Recent changes may allow for this approach. The modification of EHA, which is now referred to as IDEA (Individuals With Disabilities Act), includes diagnostic categories for students with autism and traumatic brain injury. At first, this seems the most advantageous way to go, since it begins by recognizing that this is a special group of students. However, those of us who have worked in a pediatric brain injury facility realize that educational programming for these students is tremendously complicated by their diversity of skills and behaviors.

There is no easy solution. The purpose of this manual is to educate those who will be providing services to this group of children regardless of the administrative plan. The primary author and the contributors to this book have been involved with regular education, as well as specialized treatment for brain injury. In this way, we understand both perspectives, and have set forth to provide a comprehensive view of the issues involved.

Dana S. DeBoskey, Ph.D.
Certified Teacher
Licensed School Psychologist
Licensed Psychologist

I. INTRODUCTION

In order to provide quality educational services to students with brain injury, it is important for all school personnel to understand this unique disability. This applies equally to all levels, from the superintendent of education to the regular classroom teacher. This is not a specialty that one leaves to a specific designated teacher.

Students with brain injury are found in every niche within the educational system. More often than not, they are not even recognized as brain injured unless some astute diagnostician does a thorough history with the parents and discovers information that suggests a minor or greater injury to the brain. It is easy to identify the child who has been in a brain injury rehabilitation facility for three months, but not as easy to recognize the adolescent who was unconscious for two hours after being hit by a baseball at age eight. This latter child was deemed to have lasting problems by the neurologist who obtained a normal EEG and CT scan. The parents, wanting to believe that there was no permanent damage, have probably even forgotten to mention this incident unless specifically asked by someone gathering background information for the child's current behavior problems.

The readers of this manual are provided with methods of identification, knowledge pertinent to the specific area, and strategies for intervention. The underlying basis is that damage to the brain during a child's life can lead to the presentation of issues that interfere with learning. Although the symptoms may be similar to those presented by children with developmental problems, it is necessary to understand the origin in order to properly address the needs of students who are brain injured.

Sections of this manual cover the cognitive, academic, and behavioral issues following brain injury and provide practical techniques for remediation within the educational setting. Helpful hints for teachers are offered in relation to the emotional responses they may be having to these students. Last, but certainly <u>not</u> least, is a section on preparing these students for a vocation - functioning in the outside world. Educational efforts are only as effective as their ability to prepare students for entering the community as productive and adjusted individuals.

II. EVALUATING AND DIAGNOSING

Specific criteria are set forth for all special education programs in order to qualify for the services. In most cases, these criteria can be documented by internal personnel including a variety of evaluators. In a few select categories, such as physically handicapped, a physician's prescription is required before entrance into that program is complete. Since brain injury is a physical manifestation, it seems quite possible that a physician's statement may be an integral part in formulating a special category for these students. On the surface, this way seems quite natural to an educator, but this whole issue is fraught with complications.

Another individual who would most likely be involved in brain injury cases is a neuropsychologist. Most school systems do not hire or have appropriate slots for psychologists trained in this special area. Again, one would have to rely on purchasing this service outside of the system until effective provisions could be made to have this offered through the school psychology departments. This chapter will make an effort to delineate what these "outside" personnel have to offer, as well as to consider the complexities involved in effectively evaluating and diagnosing the brain injured.

Medical Input

Which Doctor?

There are a number of specialty areas in the medical field involved in diagnosing and treating brain injury patients. In the initial stages, there is often someone from the general field of neurology. If the child required surgery, a **neurosurgeon** may be the one following the course of recovery. If surgery was not an issue, the individual involved would probably be a **neurologist**. If serious behavior problems have been evident, a **neuropsychiatrist** may be the major treating physician. If the student received rehabilitation efforts, he may be followed by a physician specializing in **physical medicine and rehabilitation**, often called a **physiatrist.**

Now that the diagnostic category of traumatic brain injury (TBI) has been introduced, there will probably be some efforts to have various physicians involved in the diagnosis process. Because of the physical nature of the injury, this procedure makes sense. However, there will be difficulties with almost any set of physicians who are chosen, primarily due to the varied experience they may have had with the brain injured population. It will not be difficult to diagnose a child who has been in a coma for a week or more; however, the diagnosis will be less clear if a child has been unconscious for 1-2 hours and there are no physical tests that document a physiological basis for neurological impairment.

Which Tests?

There are a variety of physiological tests that physicians use to determine the location and severity of injury to the brain:

1. <u>CT Scan (Computerized Axial Tomography)</u>
   The CT (or CAT) scanner is a large machine with x-ray projectors arranged in a circle. The child's head is placed in the center and x-rays are taken from various angles. A computer analyzes the pictures and gives the doctor a picture of the brain. The CT scan is useful in identifying large areas of bleeding or large contusions, but it is not a perfect picture or foolproof. A normal CT scan does <u>not</u> mean that there is nothing physically wrong with the student's brain. On the contrary, a

child who has received a brain injury due to lack of oxygen may have a normal or nearly normal CT brain scan. Thus, if the doctor sees something in the CT scan, we know there is something wrong; but if nothing is seen, we cannot be sure that the brain is completely normal.

2. MRI (Magnetic Resonance Imaging)
   The MRI gives a more detailed view of the brain than the CT scan. It is not useful early in the injury since it does not demonstrate bleeding in the early stages. It uses a strong magnetic force and does not use radiation. The MRI can identify smaller and more subtle brain anomalies or differences than the CT scan.

3. PET (Positron Emission Tomography)
   The PET scanner is a new technique used to measure some of the energy processing functions of the brain. Certain chemicals used by the brain, such as glucose (sugar), are "tagged" and the brain's ability to use them is studied with the PET scanner.

4. EEG (Electroencephalogram)
   The EEG is another test of brain function. It measures the electrical activity of the brain and compares the readings in various settings such as awake and sleeping. It is often used to verify the presence of seizure activity if this diagnosis is in question. Like the CT scan, it is better used for supportive information than for ruling out brain dysfunction. Thus, if abnormalities show up in the EEG, this means something is amiss; yet the absence of abnormalities does not mean that the brain functions in a normal manner.

   Abnormal EEGs are found in a variety of children who would not appropriately be labelled brain injured. For example, research shows that a significant number of learning disabled children show slow wave activity in the temporal-parietal area. Other groups of children with abnormal EEGs can be those with hyperactivity or attention deficit disorder.

Physicians today have a wide variety of tests to use to assist with determining the presence of brain injury. Although these can be useful for diagnostic purposes, we cannot allow the existence of abnormality on these tests to be a definitive criterion for labelling a child as brain injured. A student may show no abnormalities on most physiological testing, but still show notable learning and/or behavioral problems following an insult to the brain. A neuropsychological evaluation can help to define these more subtle issues, as well as provide information for educational planning. Placement for these children cannot be determined solely on the medical input.

Neuropsychological Input

What is a Neuropsychologist?

Within the area of psychology, there are a variety of specialty areas. A **clinical psychologist** is especially trained to evaluate, diagnose, and treat mental disorders in children and adults. A **school psychologist** has specialized training in evaluating and diagnosing children and adolescents, along with training in educational programming and curriculum development. Both of these types of psychologists are able to address most of the needs of school age children. However, when it comes to students with brain injury, it is necessary to have the input of a **neuropsychologist**. The neuropsychologist may also be a clinical or school psychologist, but has received additional training in the area of brain behavior/relationships. This specialty requires further study of neuroanatomy, physiological psychology, and expertise in a group of tests that are neuropsychological in nature.

The field of psychology is relatively new compared to other areas. When the veterans returned from WWII, the veteran hospitals were full of men who had documented injury to the brain. People like Ward Halstead and Ralph Reitan began to develop and/or fine-tune tests that would measure brain functioning of these injured veterans. These tests were not medical in nature, such as the EEG, but rather paper and pencil tasks or tests of motor activities that provided information about a person's behavioral functioning. When these results were correlated with the medical reports, various conclusions could be made about the integrity of certain portions of the brain. Through years of research, normative data have resulted whereby a psychologist trained in the area of neuropsychology can address brain functioning.

Another important issue, particularly in light of the new TBI category, is to be sure that the neuropsychologist has training and expertise in evaluating children. A person can have excellent neuropsychological skills, but, lacking significant experience with children, the applicability of the evaluation may be in question. These will be issues that school systems will need to address as they determine where and how they will be obtaining their neuropsychological information.

What is a Neuropsychological Evaluation?

As in many other fields, the specialty of neuropsychology has a number of varying viewpoints on the tests that are used to determine a child's neuropsychological status. In the main, there are three major camps. One group follows the teachings of Luria. In general, they administer what is called the Luria-Nebraska Neuropsychological Battery. A second group is led by Ralph

Reitan, and they typically give the Halstead-Reitan Neuropsychological Battery. A third group follows a process testing approach, and they take their theoretical lead from Edith Kaplan and Muriel Lezak. Oftentimes a neuropsychologist will do the Luria-Nebraska or Halstead-Reitan and supplement these batteries with tests that address specific processes. Moreover, the process approach batteries typically include various subtests that are considered part of the Luria or Reitan.

In general, no one battery should be consistently considered superior. Instead, the important component is the experience of the neuropsychologist administering the tests. It is most important, above and beyond expertise in neuropsychology, that the evaluator understand children with brain injury and be able to translate the neuropsychological information into practical use for educational systems.

In spite of the differences in these approaches, the information presented in the evaluation report is similar in nature. General areas are addressed in each, including intellectual abilities, academics, memory, learning, visual-spatial skills, language, motor skills, executive functioning, personality, and psychosocial abilities. Each of these areas will be discussed with a brief description of the types of tests that are included.

Intellectual Abilities

A standardized IQ test is a part of any comprehensive neuropsychological battery. It is very important to have this score in order to determine the significance of the other deficit areas. For example, you may have an adolescent who scores in the borderline range of IQ with a full scale score of 71. Since this score is two standard deviations below the mean, a process problem would have to be at least three standard deviations or more below to be considered significant. If you did not have this point of comparison and you assume average intelligence, you would be attributing neuropsychological deficits that may in fact be related only to lower IQ.

It is also important here to bring up the issue of what this IQ score represents for the child who is brain injured. If a student has had a severe brain injury, the IQ will likely be compromised. If the brain injury is mild or moderate in nature, the IQ score (after a year of more) may be fairly close to the premorbid (pre-injury) level. The reason for this is that an intelligence test is a measure of old learning, and it is mostly the new learning skills that are affected with brain injury.

Last, if the injury occurred very early in life, it is possible that the child has faulty learning patterns and has not been able to process new information. As the child gets older and older, the inability to learn may reduce that IQ score since information is not being acquired at the expected age level.

Academics

A general measure of word recognition, spelling, and written arithmetic skills is usually included in the evaluation. Again, the results depend upon the time since injury and the severity of the case. If the child was injured at age three or four, we can assume that the mainstream of learning has been affected, and acquisition of academic skills may be at a reduced rate over time. Thus, by the time this student reaches adolescence, the academic scores may be depressed in relation to measured ability.

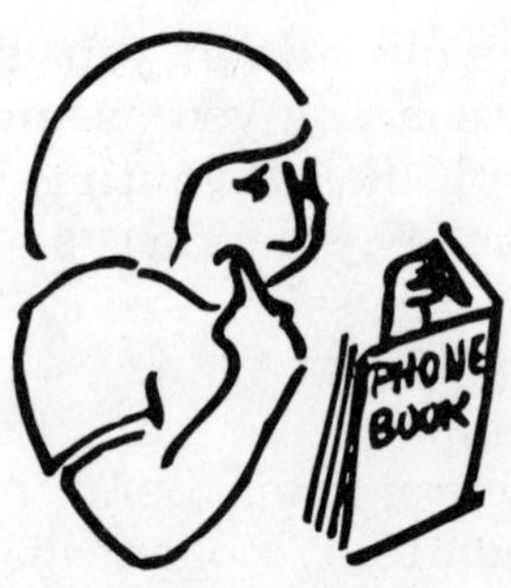

The opposite of this occurs when an adolescent is injured. Joe, a fifteen year old, received a moderate brain injury and returned to school about three months after the accident. Test results for IQ and academic levels were slightly reduced at first, but his IQ was back to 108 by the time he was tested in the school system (9 months post injury), and his standard scores for the academics were all above 100. Nevertheless, Joe was having difficulty in class absorbing new information, as well as displaying inadequate attention and concentration. His teachers believed he was having problems processing information he was hearing, similar to what happens with a learning disabled child. Joe could not qualify for the LD classes, since there was no discrepancy between his IQ (old learning) and his academic scores (also representing past learned skills). In the past, the school had to either allow Joe to experience failure in the regular classroom or try to qualify him for the behavioral program. At times, an individual would have to wait until behavior problems developed from the frustration of <u>not</u> learning before being assigned to a special class. Hopefully, this will not be the case with better understanding of TBI.

Memory

The area of memory should be examined very carefully in a neuropsychological evaluation. **Remote memory** is rarely affected. This would be long-term memories, such as what happened two or three years ago or longer. **Immediate memory** is the ability to repeat back immediately after hearing or seeing the information. **Delayed memory** is the ability to repeat back after some time has passed. In the student who is brain injured, both immediate and delayed memory will be affected.

Testing addresses both visual and auditory memory to determine if the student has a stronger channel for learning. The issue of interference is also tested, whereby the child is faced with a memory task after having an interfering event follow the memory presentation. This helps determine how much structure or stimulus-free environment is needed for effective retention of information.

Visual-Spatial Skills

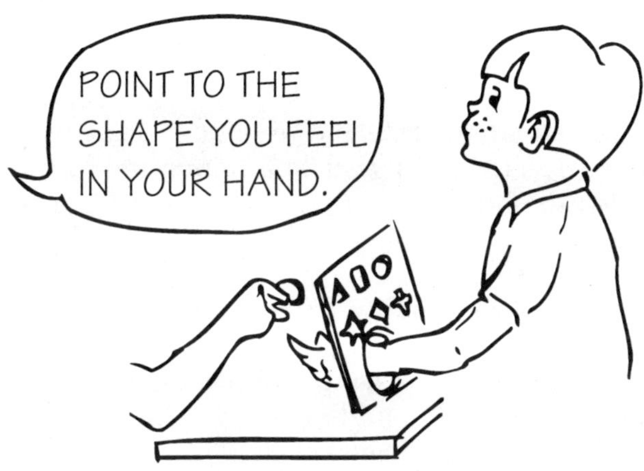

Students are tested on simple visual discrimination or matching tasks, as well as more complex issues such as subtle facial expressions. The students are shown cut-up pictures to see if they can determine what they are in order to test visual synthesis and analysis. Older students are evaluated on map skills using the United States map or their state map.

Language

This section of tests addresses the manner in which students express themselves, both verbally and in written form. A test of confrontation naming examines word retrieval problems. Verbal fluency is evaluated. A story written in response to a picture stimulus provides measurement of abstraction, grammatical skills, spelling, and creativity.

Motor Skills

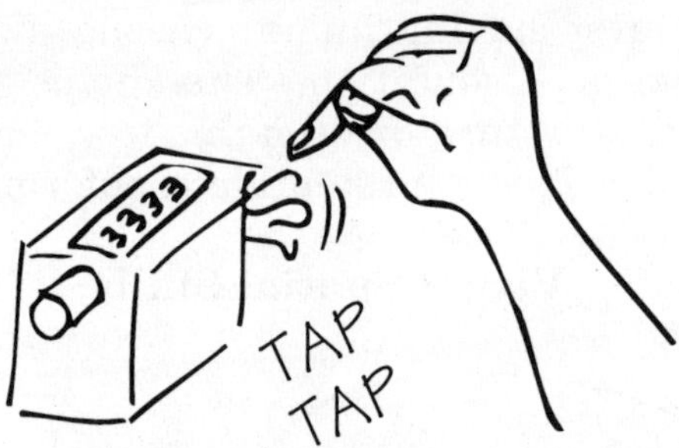

Speed and dexterity of motor responses are evaluated. The right and left hands are compared in order to shed light on asymmetry of brain functioning.

Executive Functioning

This area of testing applies more readily to adolescents since it addresses the integrity of the frontal lobes. The frontal area of the brain does not totally mature until adolescence. Therefore, tests specifically addressing the issues of conforming to task, inhibiting a motor response, hypothesis testing, and generalized problem-solving are looked at closely after age 15.

Executive functioning is a most important area to consider when students who are brain injured are starting to look at their vocational and future academic careers. The issues of college or further vocational training after high school are best answered by examining performance on the tests of executive functioning, along with a thorough work/vocational evaluation as described in Chapter 10.

Psychosocial/Personality

There are frequently behavior and/or personality changes following a brain injury. These are discussed in detail in Chapter 8. In order to determine the major areas of concern, the neuropsychologist obtains information from objective personality measures, along with behavioral reports from teachers, family, and friends.

For those of you who evaluate children with learning disabilities, language difficulties, or other specialty problems, many of the tests are similar to, or actually identical to, those used in your assessments. In many instances, the only difference is that the neuropsychologist is looking at the performance from a brain functioning perspective as opposed to a total focus on educational planning. In order for the evaluation to be the most advantageous to the school system, it is helpful for the neuropsychologist to actually come from the school psychology department, or for the testing to be administered by a neuropsychologist who is familiar with school programs and curriculum development.

III. BRAIN FUNCTION AND DYSFUNCTION

The purposes of the evaluative techniques described in Chapter 2 are to delineate if the brain is functioning within normal limits and, if not, what areas are affected. In order to better understand the evaluative processes, it is important to review both normal brain function and brain dysfunction due to brain injury. For ease of understanding, the material in this chapter is presented in a nontechnical manner. If you would like more detailed explanations, consult books in the areas of neuropsychology, neurology, and others that specifically address brain injury. Several of these are listed in the bibliography.

Normal Brain Functioning

The brain is the command center for the entire body. In addition to monitoring sensations and physical functions, it is the center of our thought processes. It is the part of the Central Nervous System (CNS) that receives and deciphers information, formulates a response, and coordinates the response through body movements. Information enters a student's body through a multitude of nerve endings. Messages are sent from the nerves to the CNS at the spinal cord. The information is transmitted up the spinal cord, through the brain stem, into the thalamus, and then into the cortex. The cortex is made up of billions of neurons or brain cells that process the information. Then messages from the cortex go back down through the same general areas from which they originated. The cerebellum is the part of the brain responsible for coordinating voluntary muscle movement and, in this respect, helps determine the appropriate motor response. The motor nerves exit from the spinal cord and carry out commands from the brain.

The brain can be divided into two halves or hemispheres. The left hemisphere of the brain controls the right side of the body, and the right hemisphere controls the left. If a student receives a severe blow to the right hemisphere of the brain, it is very likely that there will be problems with movement, feeling, and sight on the left side of the body.

The two hemispheres of the brain process information in very different manners. In a right-handed student, the left hemisphere is generally dominant, and the language function is controlled in the left brain. The left hemisphere learns by processing information in a step-by-step or linear fashion. Educators will recognize this as the sequential approach to learning. In the area of teaching reading, this is exemplified by the phonetic approach to word recognition. In the area of following directions, students with stronger left hemispheres would do best if given commands in an auditory sequential manner. For example, if someone asks you how to get somewhere in town, do you give them step-by-step auditory instructions or do you immediately draw them a little map? If you offer the sequential directions, you are tapping into left hemisphere functioning.

On the other hand, if you immediately draw a map, you may be someone who processes information more effectively in a simultaneous manner. The right brain learns by grasping multiple concepts of the bigger picture at one time. Students who learn best through this mode need to have all the information before they totally understand the issue. In the area of reading, they are those students who approach and recognize more by sight or by configuration or reading in context.

Each of the two hemispheres of the brain is divided into four major lobes. Although the brain is a very complex organism, some statements can be made about the general functioning of each lobe. **Frontal lobes** are involved with emotional control, impulse control, social function, expressive language, and voluntary movements. It is here that general problem-solving and goal setting abilities are housed. These abilities are also referred to as "executive functions," and are specifically addressed in the neuropsychological testing described in the preceding chapter. The frontal lobes do not reach maturity until adolescence or puberty.

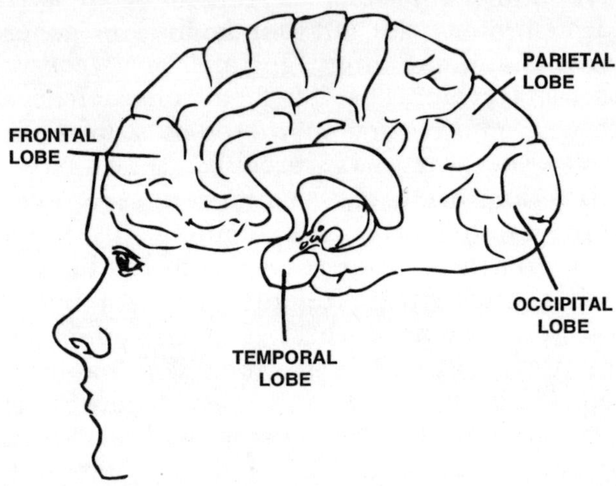

Temporal lobes are involved with memory and sequencing in general. The left temporal lobe addresses receptive language, and the right temporal lobe deals with musical awareness. **Parietal lobes** are involved with sensation. The left parietal deals with the coordination of academic skills, such as reading, and the interaction between receptive and expressive language. The right parietal is involved with awareness of spatial relationships, recognition of faces, time awareness, judgment, and awareness of the significance of things that have occurred. **Occipital lobes** are involved with reception and perception of the visual image.

The dominant left hemisphere controls verbal abilities such as language, comprehension, reading, talking, and writing. The right hemisphere controls visual-spatial functions such as copying, drawing, visual memory, rhythm, and musical appreciation.

Brain Dysfunction

Injury to the brain can occur in a variety of different ways. Although a blow to the head (closed head or open head injury) is probably the most common occurrence, brain injuries also result from strokes, tumors, lack of oxygen, or some type of infection process. All of these conditions will now be addressed in greater detail.

Closed Head Injury

When a child receives a blow to the head that does not break the skull, the brain vibrates back and forth within the unbroken skull. Since the skull does not give, the brain bangs up against the bony side of the skull, causing bruising and shearing of the axons (cores of the nerve fibers). This procedure results in what is called generalized diffuse damage to both hemispheres.

The severity of this injury can vary from a mild concussion where the child is only dazed or confused to a severe injury where the child is in a coma for weeks or even months. Brain injuries are rated as mild, moderate, and severe, using both length of unconsciousness and a rating scale called the Glasgow Coma Scale. This rating scale was developed to more clearly define the phenomenon of coma. A child can be considered to be in a comatose state even if not completely unconscious.

In recent years, the effects of what had been considered insignificant brain injuries in the past are now being taken into consideration for diagnosis of learning problems and educational planning. As has been mentioned earlier, a thorough history of a child who is having learning and/or behavioral problems may reveal an injury that medical personnel have heretofore attributed with little to no significance. Such injuries may include a fall off a horse, a tumble down the basement stairs, or a hard tackle in football at age twelve. What is even more significant is a history that reveals a series of these types of incidents with the same child. Research is showing that the effects of more than one mild brain injury is really multiplicative in nature, so that children may experience more significant deficits from a second blow to the head than would normally occur if there had not been a prior injury.

Open Head Injury

An open head injury occurs when a child receives a blow that either penetrates the skull, such as with a knife or gunshot wound, or when the skull is fractured due to the focal and severe impact to one area of the skull. Many people feel that this type of injury has to be worse since there are obvious physical signs of damage. This, however, is not necessarily the case. For example, damage from a knife will lead to severe problems in the specific area of penetration, but the brain does not experience the pervasive problems resulting from the diffuse generalized damage of the closed head injury.

Stroke

Although generally occurring in the much older population, a very small percentage of children experience hemorrhaging in the brain. This can lead to generalized brain injury by the irritant effect of blood in the affected areas of the brain. Although similar, the cognitive and behavioral changes are not exactly like that of a closed head injury.

Tumor

Tumors can occur at all ages. Sometimes a tumor will be present in a child but not diagnosed until later years. If discovered at an early age, surgery may be initiated. The type of damage is generally focal in nature. The brain tissue that has been replaced by the tumor has most likely been severely compromised. There can also be damage from the entry into the brain to remove the tumor.

Lack of Oxygen

Anoxic (or hypoxemic) brain injury is another type of generalized damage that can occur in children. It is caused by a lack of blood flow to the brain - depriving the brain of oxygen and nutrients vital for its survival. Stopping blood flow to the brain for over three minutes causes brain damage, while stopping blood flow for ten minutes can cause brain death. This is most common in children who have suffered a near drowning, a cardiac arrest or a respiratory arrest. This can occur at birth if the cord is wrapped around the baby's neck. Anoxic brain injury can also occur along with traumatic brain injury. It is most common where there is massive blood loss, injury to the lungs, or such severe swelling in the brain that blood flow into the brain is seriously reduced. Anoxic brain injury affects deep brain structures and results in problems with memory, sensation, coordination, and vision.

Infectious Processes

Brain injury occurs when children contact infectious diseases such as meningitis or encephalitis. The extent of the cognitive and behavioral problems is, of course, related to the severity of the case. The brain is affected in a diffuse fashion, so that generally both hemispheres are affected. As educators, you will find that some parents do not even mention that their children had such a disease unless specifically asked. This generally occurs when the case has been mild in nature, and the parents either were not told or did not understand the probable residual effects.

IV. BACKGROUND INFORMATION FOR A VARIETY OF EDUCATORS

There is a wide range of variability in almost any specialized group of children; however, the brain injured population presents one of the greatest diversities. For this reason, it is especially important that all groups of educators understand the characteristics and needs of these students. In spite of Traumatic Brain Injury (TBI) now being included as a separate special education category, some of these children can be appropriately served in a regular classroom or another special education category. Thus, the following chapter provides all educational personnel with information that is important to their particular area.

School Psychologists and Other Evaluators

School psychologists with specialized training in neuropsychology should already have adequate information about this group of children. They will be a part of the specialized team that will finalize the appropriate evaluation and placement. However, school psychologists who are not specifically trained, as well as other evaluators such as educational diagnosticians or speech pathologists, will provide a screening service for further evaluation. For this reason, it is very important that these "screeners" understand the salient issues so that children will not fall through the cracks or be inappropriately placed.

The school psychologist should be astutely aware of findings in the psychological data that suggest and/or document neurological impairment, particularly if the injury is one that is not readily identifiable from a physical standpoint. Obtaining a thorough history from the parents is important. Many times injured students will return to school with the assumption that there will be minimal residual effects. The parents may be able to clarify or substantiate subtle changes that indicate a potential need for special services, whereas the students themselves will probably deny that there are any problems.

In reviewing the psychological data, signs of possible problems would be similar to those seen in learning disabled children, with a wide range of inconsistencies that include both intra and inter subtest scatter. There will very likely be processing difficulties that may or may not meet the guidelines for a learning disability category. If the injury is recent, there will not be a major discrepancy between ability (IQ) and achievement (academic testing), again nullifying a diagnosis of Specific Learning Disability (SLD).

Another important issue for the school psychologist to consider is that of behavioral problems in this population. Unless these students have had emotional problems prior to the injury, the etiology of their behavioral issues are very different from students who are generally delinquent or purposefully manipulative in nature. Students who are brain injured often "act before they think," and therefore do not have a purposeful agenda to their inappropriate behavior. It stands to reason that appropriate interventions must take this difference into account. Even though the behaviors may be identical to the casual observer, their origin necessitates a behavioral approach that allows for the lack of impulse control.

It is important for educational diagnosticians to realize that a lack of deficit in academic functioning does not negate the fact that students who are brain injured are having learning problems. We must remember that the academic scores typically obtained are a measure of "old learning." Because of this, it might be very appropriate for evaluators to add a "new learning" task to their battery of tests.

For the speech pathologist evaluating neurologically impaired students, it is helpful to have sufficient knowledge of the differences between developmental disorders and those that are more likely due to organic deficits. In this way, a speech therapy program can best address the specific needs of this population.

Supervisors of these evaluators should provide continuous inservice programs relevant to the assessment of neurologically impaired students. This is a field where there is constant change and revision. There is a continual need for updated educational efforts.

Staffing Specialists

Titles may vary from state to state, but these individuals are educators who coordinate and oversee the placement of students into appropriate special programs. It is important that they clearly understand the diversity of students who are brain injured. Each case must be looked at with placement considerations based on a multitude of factors - not just meeting the county guidelines or criteria. It may be that the brain injured student's needs can best be met through a combination of two programs, even though this is not typically done. The staffing specialist will have schools resist placements that go beyond the ordinary. It will be the job of this specialist to educate the personnel in that particular school so that they can understand the need for flexibility. In order to feel confident and comfortable, these specialists must be knowledgeable in the special characteristics of these students. Chapters 5, 6, and 8 will be most helpful in formulating a knowledge base regarding children who are brain injured.

Principals

The principal sets the stage for the general attitude held by the personnel in that school. Since flexibility is an important characteristic in helping to educate this group of children, it is vital for the principal to support a potentially creative curriculum plan. It will also be helpful for this school leader to thoroughly understand the etiology of the behavior problems exhibited by children with brain injury. A principal is often the ultimate manager of discipline, and it may be necessary for this person to make some concessions in certain individual cases.

Curriculum Specialists

Students who are brain injured often have trouble with memory and new learning. Thus, the curriculum must provide opportunities to learn the same issues over and over in different contexts so that these students can master the skill to the automatic level. Opportunities for repetition are mandatory and should be included in all subject areas.

Guidance Counselors

It is important that guidance counselors thoroughly understand both the cognitive and behavioral characteristics of this population. When students who are brain injured require advice on schedule of classes, it is helpful to know their cognitive deficits. In this way, a counselor can provide the most appropriate guidance regarding the level of difficulty of classes, as well as be looking at a potential college major or vocational career.

If students with brain injury are referred for behavioral difficulties, it is imperative that the counselor understand brain injury issues. Significant deficits in frontal lobe functioning or problem solving will require a specialized intervention strategy that will allow for these cognitive effects. Memory may also be a factor contributing to a behavioral problem. The counselor will want to provide ways in which these students can be cued by either a teacher or self-cuing techniques.

Teachers

As we have emphasized throughout this manual, the diversity of students with brain injury requires that all types of teachers have a working knowledge of this group. Students with brain injury can be appropriately placed in a wide variety of settings.

Regular Classroom

In keeping with maintaining the least recidivistic environment, regular classroom teachers will find that they must understand how to interact with this population. It is very important that children with brain injury have appropriate role models, and this is most readily available in the regular classes. Teachers must keep in mind that these students may be different in the way they approach either academic tasks or interaction with others. If educators can be flexible in allowing for these differences, this group will have the chance they desperately need to interact with regularly placed students.

Specific Learning Disabilities (SLD)

Although it has not been perfect, this category has been the least offensive placement to many students and parents. Students who are brain injured often look completely "normal," both physically and mentally, and find it difficult to accept the need for specialized academic help. There have been major difficulties getting some groups of children qualified for this type of program, particularly the older student. Frequently, they will meet processing criteria due to a variation in cognitive functioning, but will not meet academic criteria. As we have mentioned previously, the academic scores are a measurement of old learning which often remains intact. This does not negate, however, that students who are brain injured typically have significant problems with learning new concepts. This learning problem can often be dealt with most effectively in the SLD classroom.

The authors would recommend that the academic criteria be waived for these students on a case by case basis. This exception would be most critical for those students who do not display other problems that qualify them for any other special programs. The new category of TBI may eventually provide an alternative, but there will still be children who could be most efficiently served in the SLD classroom.

Physically Handicapped (PH)

This category is most appropriate for the students who have been in a coma for an extended period of time and, as a result, display severe physical and cognitive limitations. When the higher functioning children are referred to this program, there is frequently resistance by parents and the students themselves to placement with others having severe deficits. If they do not have obvious physical limitations, they see themselves as very different from the majority of other classmates in this category. This resistance can prevent them from receiving maximum benefit from the program.

The PH teacher may have to make special efforts to assist the child who is brain injured in becoming part of the group. At times, these higher functioning individuals can feel important by helping those who have significantly greater physical limitations. The PH classroom, along with mainstreaming for certain classes, can be an alternative option. Again, it is hoped that the new category of TBI can offer another possible placement option. Nevertheless, there will usually be a group of severely physically limited TBI children who continue to be best served in the PH classroom, even after the TBI category is delineated in the school systems across the nation.

Mentally Handicapped (EMN, TMH, and SPMH)

Some brain injuries lead to varying degrees of compromising of intellectual abilities. Thus, when such students are tested, they may technically qualify for one of the three categories of mentally handicapped. We use the word "technically" since an IQ score of 65 can represent very different abilities depending upon the etiology of the deficiency. For example, John is a twelve year old child who was tested at age three and placed into early special education classes based upon a 65 IQ score falling with the EMH (Educably Mentally Handicapped) range. His mother had been in special education, and he had two sisters who were also in EMH classes. The etiology of John's mental deficiency was developmental in nature. His academic progress had been consistently slow throughout his school career, and his academic standard scores fell within the 60's.

Mary, on the other hand, had been an above average student, maintaining a B average throughout her six years of school. In the summer before entering seventh grade, she was thrown from her bicycle when she was hit by a truck. She remained in a coma for three months, spent six additional months in a comprehensive rehabilitation center, and was evaluated for appropriate school placement by the school psychologist. An IQ score of 65 was obtained, yet the standard scores for academics fell within the upper 80's to high 90's. Verbal IQ was compromised due to problems with language expression, and Performance IQ was down due to ataxia problems and decreased motor speed. When Mary was placed in the EMH class, she was very unhappy and said she was not retarded like the others. She was, in fact, accurate, as her "retarded" IQ score was not obtained in the same way as most of the other students.

These examples point out why placement in mentally handicapped classes may not be appropriate for a number of students who are brain injured, particularly those injured later in life. If a severe injury occurs very early, normal learning does not take place, and these students may be effectively handled in the handicapped setting.

Teachers of mentally handicapped students must be aware of the fact that students who are brain injured may not present in the same manner as the other students. A thorough review of the cognitive and behavioral deficits described in this manual will help these educators to understand some of these differences.

Emotionally Handicapped (EH)

Chapter 8 describes behavioral problems that can result from injury to the brain. Such behaviors may qualify the students for the Emotionally Handicapped (EH) program. As we have indicated previously, it is important that teachers attempting to manage these behaviors understand their origin. This realization is necessary for effective treatment planning. On the other hand, students with brain injury can also learn to manipulate in the same way as the other behaviorally disordered children. Teachers will need to learn to discriminate between those behaviors that are neurologically based and those that are learned for the purpose of controlling the environment.

Language Impaired

A large number of neurologically impaired children are found in classes that are specifically designated for language impaired students. In some school systems, there is a requirement that there be a high capability in the performance area so that this strength can be used to remediate or compensate for the language weakness. This, however, may not be the case for students with closed head injury, since they may experience diffuse difficulties to both hemispheres. At times, a combination of language impaired and SLD is effective for treating these students.

V. COGNITIVE PROCESSING NEEDS AND STRATEGIES

In order for a student to learn, information is processed through various sensory modes. Following head trauma, the manner by which a student previously processed information can be significantly affected, resulting in learning problems. Since schools play a major role in the rehabilitation of children who are brain injured, it is important to differentiate between weak and strong modes of processing so that you, as a teacher, can assist the student by teaching through the stronger modality. Learning can be facilitated by capitalizing upon the student's stronger mode, while decreasing presentation of information through the weaker mode. For example, visual learners can best be taught to read using a sight-word approach, while auditory learners can best be taught to read by blending isolated sounds into words. Another teaching technique might entail combining methods of processing, as in the VAKT (Visual, Auditory, Kinesthetic, Tactile) approach and over-cuing. By presenting the same information through the various sensory modes, an individual may be better able to comprehend and encode information.

As a result of deficits children experience following brain trauma, program development for the injured child must emphasize a process orientation. This chapter will explain the various methods of processing information, and then will review the cognitive deficits which might be observed following brain trauma and suggestions for assisting the child to learn and compensate for his impairments.

Methods of Processing Information

Visual/Auditory/Kinesthetic/ Tactile Processing

Children learn through the sensory modalities. These methods are almost self-explanatory by their names. Visual processing involves the student seeing the information, such as a diagram presented on the blackboard or in a textbook. Auditory processing involves information which a student hears, such as a classroom lecture presented by the teacher. Kinesthetic and tactile processing involves learning through movement and touch, respectively. For example, teaching the alphabet by having a student repeatedly feel and trace a wooden letter combines these two types of processing. The VAKT approach to learning combines all four of these senses. For example, the word is presented visually to the student, the student is required to say the word, and at the same time trace an example of the wood with his finger. This multisensory approach, or simultaneous association of visual, auditory, kinesthetic, and tactile stimuli, is an effective method for enhancing learning in children with brain injury.

It is important for the teacher to have knowledge of the child's strongest mode of processing. Even unimpaired children have preferable methods for processing information. The teacher must be careful to avoid teaching exclusively to the deficit or weaker mode. Presenting information only through the auditory channel in lecturing hinders visual learners, as well as individuals with auditory processing and auditory memory problems.

If you observe a child who is brain injured consistently squinting or closing one eye when reading, "missing" when reaching for an object, or not learning information on one side of his paper, books, or the blackboard, the child is most likely having visual processing problems which need to be taken into consideration within the classroom setting. In conjunction with checking with the students and their parents regarding a recent ophthalmological evaluation, the teacher may want to be sure the students are presented with the same information through the auditory mode and the visual mode. For problems such as visual neglect, taping a note to the desk reminding the child to look to the neglected side, or taping arrows across the desk, may increase the child's ability to perceive information in that field of vision.

Sequential vs. Simultaneous Processing

A well-known researcher in the field of neuropsychology, A. Luria, proposed that information received must be processed either sequentially (in temporal order), simultaneously (as a whole gestalt), or both. Further, he hypothesized that the preferred mode of processing relates closely to the child's learning style. Although children may at times alternate between these two modes of processing, they generally have a dominant processing style. Thus, we can classify children into sequential or simultaneous processors/learners.

Sequential processors prefer input to be arranged in serial order, linearly and temporally relating an idea to the preceding idea. Two examples of tasks requiring sequential learning are included in the K-ABC (which will be discussed in a later section of this book). These tasks require the child to repeat numbers in the same order as presented auditorially by the examiner, and to reproduce in a correct order the series of hand movements made by the examiner.

Deficits in a child's ability to sequentially process information can occur following head trauma, and these could be evidenced by the child's decreased ability to understand the chronology of historical events, difficulty using appropriate steps for science experiments or stepwise procedures for solving mathematical calculations (such as borrowing or long division), failure to understand rules in a game, inability to comprehend and follow oral directions, deficiencies in decoding and phonetic spelling, and difficulty recalling the sequential order of events in reading.

Simultaneous processors prefer input to be integrated and synthesized simultaneously. They want to see the whole picture before producing an appropriate solution. They accomplish this through processing several stimuli at once, rather than stimulus-by-stimulus. Examples of tasks requiring simultaneous processing on the K-ABC consist of requiring the child to recall spatial locations of stimuli, identify objects pictured in partially completed drawings, and construction of a novel design from several geometric figures.

Brain trauma resulting in simultaneous processing deficits can be detected in a child having difficulty understanding the main idea of a story, decreased comprehension of the meaning of paragraphs, and difficulty understanding more complex mathematical principles, and can result in rote learning without a clear understanding of a concept. In simultaneous processing, the child must be able to integrate various aspects of a problem in order to solve the problem with maximum efficiency. Missing a portion of the problem affects the child's ability to formulate a correct response.

When attempting to provide children with assistance through educational remediation following head trauma, remediation techniques must be matched to the child's strengths in mental processing and preferred learning style. Following head trauma, the child's premorbid learning style and resultant processing deficits must be considered in order to enhance the child's learning capacity.

Input vs. Output

As you begin to review evaluations and notes in regard to a child's rehabilitation following brain injury, terms such as input and output will be encountered. Input relates to perception. It is the child's ability to receive information in the environment. Information is then processed, organized (or encoded) and placed in short-term memory storage. Deficits in any of a child's senses or in attention/concentration can affect the taking in (input) of information. Given this definition of input, output refers to the expression of information, either through a verbal or nonverbal response. Speech/language deficits and motor involvement following brain trauma affect the student's output or ability to make a correct response. In assessing output difficulties, remember that these problems may actually reflect input difficulties. If information is not properly taken in, the response will be affected.

Encoding vs. Retrieval

Encoding refers to the manner in which the child organizes information that is taken in. The process is analogous to a filing system. When children process information, they place the information in a file. When required to make a response based upon that information, they search the memory bank for that file and pull out the necessary information. Frequently, a child who is brain injured loses the ability to effectively organize (encode) the information. Information taken in does not always get into the proper file. When required to retrieve (find) the information, it is not in the proper file, or is scattered throughout various files, making the response inadequate or incorrect.

Retrieval refers to the process of getting information from storage. As with the input and output relationship, the same is true of the encoding and retrieval relationship. The child's capacity to consolidate and retrieve information is critical in scholastic performance. If information is not input, processed or encoded properly, retrieval will be affected.

The various models of processing information which we have just discussed can be viewed on a continuum.

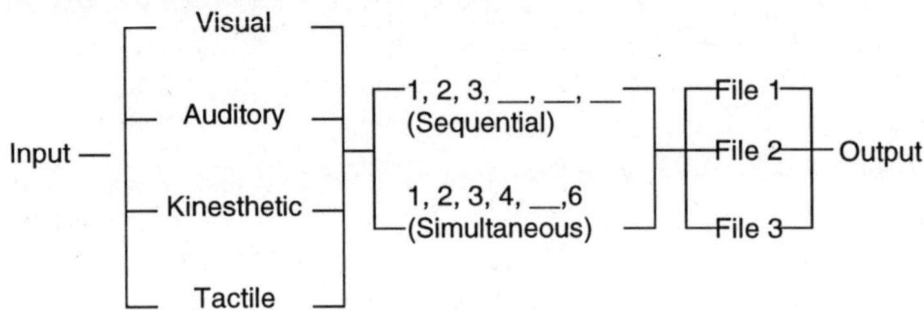

Information is taken in through visual, auditorial, kinesthetic, and tactile modes. It is processed sequentially or simultaneously and encoded (organized). When a teacher asks a question, the child goes to one of the files, retrieves information, and makes a response.

Cognitive Deficits

While processing deficits can significantly affect the child's ability to learn, cognitive deficits associated with brain trauma need to be identified and addressed with the same degree of concern in the classroom setting.

Attention/Concentration

Almost all neurologically impaired children display attention/concentration deficits. Children who are brain injured have significant difficulty focusing and sustaining attention over time and are highly distractible.

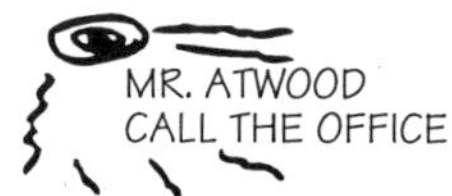

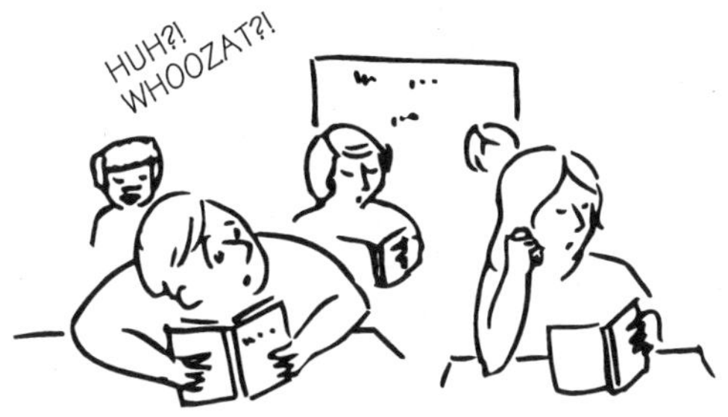

Attention/concentration refers to the amount of time that a child remains on-task. Attention usually refers to a brief period of time, while concentration is the ability to sustain attention over time. Attention can be as brief as the amount of time required for a child to recognize or perceive information, or as long as the time required to process information presented in a 2-3 hour lecture. Selective attention deficits result in children being unable to focus attention on meaningful information. For example, the child may appear to be sitting and attentive to a lecture. In fact, instead of processing the information the teacher is presenting, the child is thinking of a football game to be played after school.

Since attention and memory are fundamental components of learning, deficits in these areas lead to significant academic problems, particularly in assimilating new information. Other effects of decreased attention/concentration that the teacher may observe in the brain injured child's classroom performance are distractibility, difficulty following instructions, inability to manage two or more steps in one task simultaneously, and inability to shift attention. This decreased ability for the child to shift his attention may result in perseveration (continuing to exhibit the same behavior or make the same verbal response, despite a change in the task/question). The student continues to count (as he was doing in a previous classroom assignment), even when a new activity requires him to categorize objects and make a verbal response.

Interventions for Attention/ Concentration Deficits:

1. Control distractors in the classroom which can cause lapses in attention.

2. Use environmental manipulations, such as placing the child's desk near the teacher's desk, in the front of the room, or in an area where he is not surrounded by other children, particularly more active children who may distract him.

3. Shift activities fairly frequently, but allow the child time and assistance to get started on the new task.

4. Provide the child with frequent breaks, particularly following academically and cognitively demanding activities. The adolescent and young adult who is brain injured should be assisted to choose classes in a manner which would optimize their attention. For example, breaks or study halls should be scheduled between academically demanding classes. Remember, students who are brain injured may fatigue more readily than other students, thus their tolerance levels and "overloading" need to be considerations in the educational setting.

5. Encourage older students to use a tape recorder in the classroom so they can review lectures and compensate for "missing" information.

6. When presenting a student with a new assignment, ask the student to repeat instructions before beginning the task. Then provide him with a checklist to be filled out as he completes each step of the task. Time limits next to each step can assist the student to self-monitor when required to complete tasks independently.

7. Redirect the student's attention as soon as you observe lapses in concentration.

8. For small children, game playing can be used to increase attention. Games allow children to "practice" attending to one task. At first, games should be fairly short, but length should be increased as the child demonstrates improvements.

9. Use behavior management techniques to gradually increase attention. Provide the child with reinforcement and praise following successful attention to a task for a specified time frame. Initially, provide the child with close supervision, but gradually reinforce appropriately attending to tasks as you distance yourself from the student's desk (i.e., move to another area of the room; leave the room briefly).

10. In attempting activities to increase a student's attention/concentration, the teacher must be certain to use exercises for which the child has the cognitive and academic skills to complete without assistance.

11. Assign a "listening buddy." A classmate is chosen to sit next to the impaired student to insure that being on the correct page, following along with the teacher, and taking notes is accomplished. At higher grade levels, the "buddy" could make carbon copies of notes,

which could be integrated with the notes of the student who is brain injured. This "buddy" is to provide assistance only when needed. Some families have hired aides to assist their children. The aides provide the same function as the "buddy," but they are not peers and may bring greater attention to the "different" student in the classroom, resulting in even more difficulty forming peer relationships.

Auditory and Visual Memory/Sequencing

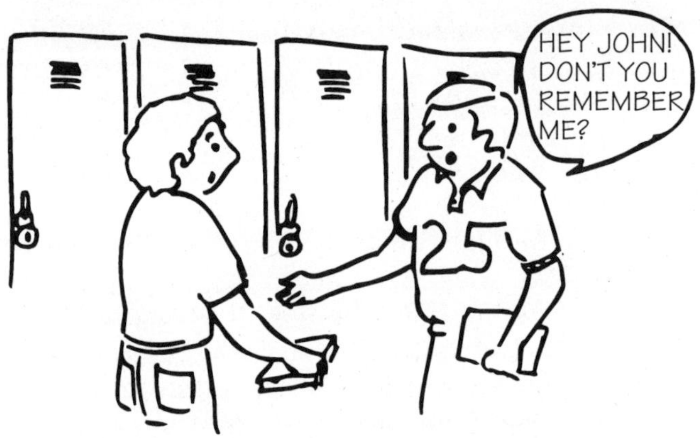

Memory impairments have been shown to be the most common cognitive deficit in pediatric brain injury cases. Almost all neurologically impaired children need training and assistance to compensate for visual and/or auditory memory problems. These residual effects are more frequently observed in short-term (day-to-day) memory. Only in severe brain trauma is long-term memory (ability to recall events before the injury) affected. Given this pattern, while the child might demonstrate average to above average intellectual skills (which are generally a measure of old learning), new learning will be a problem due to short-term memory deficits. The individual's ability to order or sequence events or information is also affected by memory deficits.

Addressing memory deficits alone is not effective in rehabilitating children who are brain injured. Weakened mechanisms underlying the impairment, such as insufficient rehearsal, susceptibility to distractors or interference, inadequate encoding abilities, visual or auditory perceptual impairments, and retrieval problems, need examination and remediation if indicated. For example, improving the student's ability to organize auditory information will improve overall recall. These underlying processes may at one time have been automatic, but they take conscious effort following the injury, since the child's brain might have lost the ability to perform the function automatically.

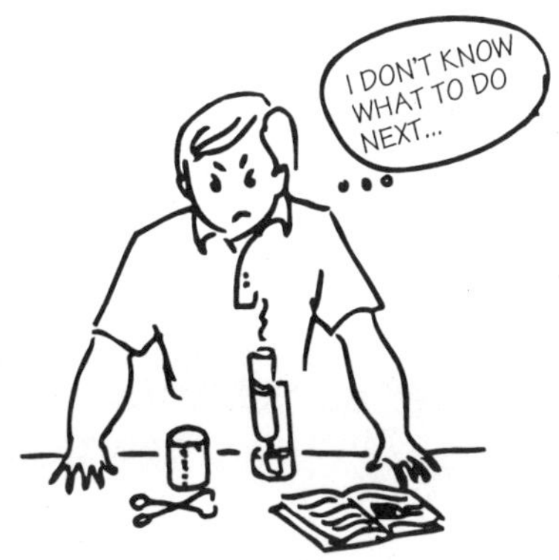

The type and steps in the mechanism processing information can be best illustrated as follows:

Registration → Processing → Encoding →
(Organizing) ↓

← ← ← ←

↓
Retention/Storage
→ Immediate → (Short & Long-Term) → Retrieval

Since learning and memory functions are less efficient following head trauma, repetition, multimodal cuing, consistency, and emphasis on generalization from one context to another are necessary. Other techniques to improve memory functions are numerous and must be based upon the student's specific deficits. A student with auditory memory deficits primarily due to encoding should be assisted to organize notes from lectures and encouraged to develop visual images to enhance recall. In contrast, a student with visual memory problems will need assistance to formulate associations between information (for example, between peoples' names and their faces) and should be encouraged to verbally mediate (talk his way through) diagrams, forming auditory associations. Individuals with encoding deficits will need cues to recall information, while those with storage problems may require specific directions presented auditorially and visually. Individuals with storage problems should not be expected to perform a new, or even fairly new, task or exercise without the directions.

Within the classroom, memory deficits can be observed in some of the following ways: difficulty with new learning, difficulty returning to an assignment or exercise following an interruption, misinterpretation, confusion, difficulty transferring newly learned information from one setting to another (the information is content bound), and inability to add on to previously learned information. For example, a student can obtain a B in Algebra II, but cannot remember how to apply the same concepts for Algebra III.

Interventions for Memory/Sequencing Deficits:

1. Encourage the student to ask for clarification of directions and write down instructions.

2. Encourage the sequence of reading directions, paraphrasing or writing them, and re-reading directions before beginning the task.

3. Provide the student with written directions or directions presented via sequential arrangement of pictures.

4. Encourage taping of lectures to be reviewed by the student at a later date.

5. Assist the student to associate information by providing associations (visual and auditory) and other ways to recall information.

6. Help the student to verbally mediate visual information and/or provide that same information auditorially.

7. Provide instructions in listening skills by using tape recorded materials and talking books in conjunction with textbooks.

8. Assist the student to develop mental pictures depicting the newly presented material.

9. Encourage pre-reading of assignments.

10. Write new assignments on the blackboard as well as providing them orally.

11. Provide instruction in small steps and require the student to check-off each step as it is completed.

12. Provide the student with a written schedule and keep this schedule as consistent as possible.

13. Encourage the use of a memory notebook which includes a list of "things to do." The student should be assisted or cued to write assignments in this notebook as soon as they are given. If the student has difficulty writing or enjoys computers, a digital diary may be more effective.

14. Frequently probe or assess the student's recall of information by using brief quizzes rather than major or cumulative exams.

15. Allow the student time to practice and review the information and present it more than one time. Repetition is a key to learning with individuals who are brain injured.

16. Encourage the student to review classroom information on a daily basis.

17. Provide the parents with a daily list of activities or new learning and encourage them to review the information with their child after school. Assist them to present the information in the same manner in which you present it in the classroom. Encourage consistency.

18. Do not assume that the student has knowledge of a previous concept when providing information which builds on that concept.

19. Use memory training games which require the child to recall the sequence of pictures, numbers, or words presented, or games which require them to recall the missing item in a set. As the child's memory improves, increase the amount of time between presentation of the stimulus (numbers, pictures, etc.) and recall, and gradually introduce distractors (unrelated activities) during the time between stimulus presentation and recall.

20. Another memory training game, "building a house," requires the student to observe and recall the number of blocks and placement of these blocks. After the teacher allows the student time to study the "house," it is knocked down and the student is asked to build the same "house."

Comprehension

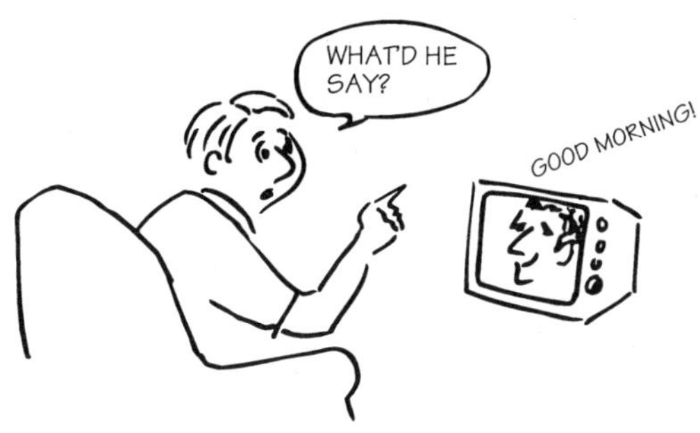

Comprehension, for the purposes of our subject matter, is defined as a student's ability to perceive and understand information seen, heard, or touched. Deficits in comprehension impede the student's ability to make sense out of the environment and can be observed in various ways within the classroom. Difficulty understanding written and pictorial directions, difficulty following conversations due to decreased understanding of vocabulary, misinterpretation of messages from books and lectures, literal interpretations of jokes and proverbs, and decreased understanding of questions are behaviors of students who are brain injured which can be indicative of comprehension problems.

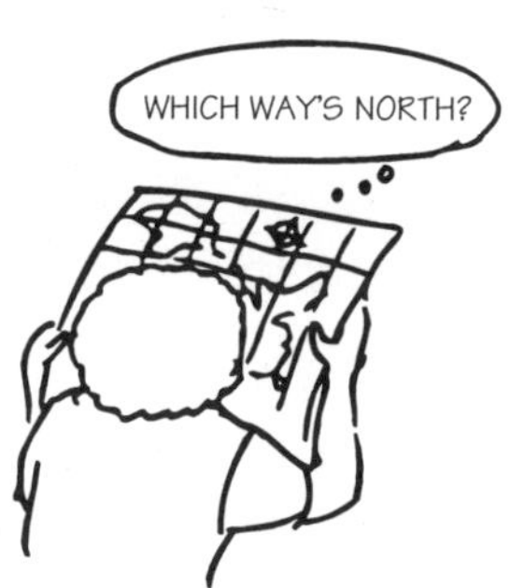

Interventions for Comprehension Deficits:

1. To improve auditory comprehension, choose a child's favorite record and request the child

to identify particular sounds that he likes/dislikes or ask him to identify similar sounds in different records.

2. Assist the child in discriminating between two very different sound patterns. As the child becomes more proficient, request him to discriminate between increasingly similar speech sounds.

3. Avoid using long explanations with children who demonstrate comprehension problems.

4. Provide auditory and visual directions which depict the same information.

5. Explain higher level vocabulary words and request the student to paraphrase directions.

6. Be certain the student understands all the questions asked.

Problem Solving

Problem solving skills fall in the realm of higher level cognitive abilities because they require a multi-step process. Any weaknesses in the steps necessary for problem solving affect the student's ability to formulate an effective problem solving strategy, initiate the problem solving process, and follow it through to completion. The child must be able to comprehend what is being asked, identify similarities and differences, analyze and synthesize, determine the process to apply to the problem, logically sequence and follow-through on the necessary problem solving steps, and compare the results (the answer) with the defined problem. Any weaknesses along the problem solving continuum will affect the child's ability to effectively problem-solve. For example, deficits in attention/concentration can affect the problem solving process. A student using an appropriate procedure will have a lapse in concentration that results in "forgetting" the strategy. This forces going through the problem solving process again in order to "get back" the appropriate technique.

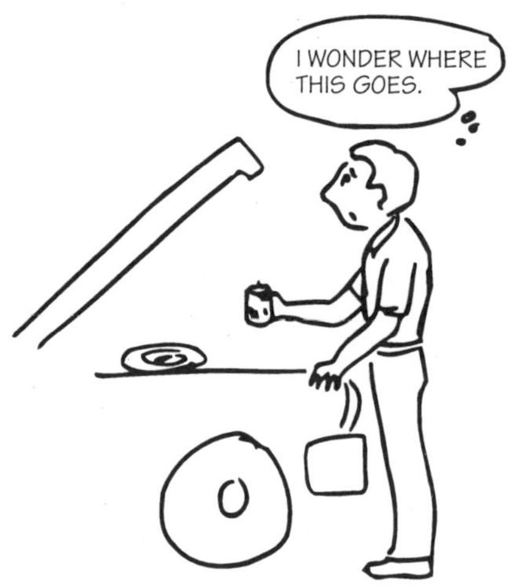

Given the complexity of the problem solving process, deficits in this area are common among students who are brain injured. Inflexibility, limitations in convergent and divergent thinking, difficulty anticipating consequences and determining cause-effect relationships, failure to plan ahead, problems in analysis/synthesis of information, and reduced creativity are signs of problem-solving deficits in a brain injured student. Students with problem-solving impairments may have difficulty completing arithmetic word problems, appear "lost" even in a familiar environment, have difficulty following the logic of games, and become more frequently involved in altercations with their classmates.

Interventions for Problem Solving Deficits:

1. Programmed learning fosters problem solving.

2. Assist the student to write out alternative solutions to problems.

3. Using comic strips that are cut and placed in an illogical order, assist the student to re-sequence the comic to result in an appropriate cause-effect relationship.

4. Pair the student with another classmate or small group for game playing involving logic.

5. During free time and after school, encourage the student and parents to play games on the computer or institute "family game" times.

6. When problem-solving, require the student to write down the materials and logical steps necessary for problem solving before attempting to work through the problem solving process.

7. A more specific technique for students having difficulties in the beginning of the problem solving process is as follows: a) require the child to match a series of pictures to identical objects; b) require the child to match objects to similar (rather than identical) objects or pictures; c) assist the child to learn to choose objects that represent a category; and d) require the child to match objects or pictures based upon their function. This technique will assist the child in the beginning of the problem solving process to discriminate relevant/irrelevant information.

Organization

Organizational skills are a higher level cognitive function. They require the integration of memory, concentration, problem-solving and sequencing abilities.

Naturally the student's ability to organize is related to some degree to his age. A young child is not expected to be organized without external structure. However, adolescents and young adults who are brain injured may require this same degree of structure to function at an optimal level.

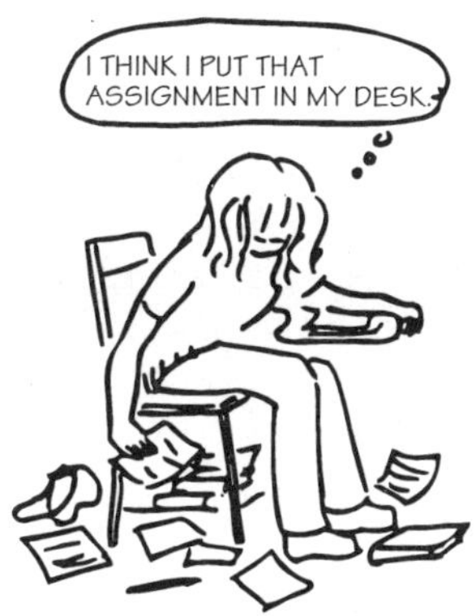

In a classroom setting, organizational problems manifest themselves in a student having difficulty summarizing, outlining, sequencing, and discriminating relevant from irrelevant information. Difficulty meeting assignment deadlines, lack of integration in written assignments, "sloppiness" (for example, a math paper with problems written all over the page, rather than in rows or columns), and lack of preparedness (forgetting to return assignments, tardiness, failing to bring a sharp pencil or pen), are further examples of disorganization which the teacher may observe in a brain injured student. It is not unusual for these students to try their hardest and still be unable to "keep it all together."

Interventions for Organization Deficits:

1. Provide external structure and consistency in the classroom.

2. Provide the student with step-by-step instructions which organize the assignment.

3. Assist the student to integrate lecture notes with textbook information.

4. Monitor the student's papers for neatness and assist him to approach assignments in an organized fashion.

5. Divide large projects into small assignments and provide the student with deadlines to complete each assignment. Be sure the student has these deadlines listed in a memory notebook. Assist the child to plan ahead in accomplishing these assignments.

6. Provide the student with a list of items needed for each class per day.

7. Provide the student with a list of assignments due each day or assist in incorporating this information in the memory notebook.

8. The older student should be encouraged to use clearly marked file folders, organizers, and a calendar for each class and classroom assignments.

9. Assist the student to develop "study schedules" to avoid "cramming" for exams.

10. In some cases, a classroom aide might be necessary to provide the student with note-taking assistance.

Motor Skills

While motor problems are usually not considered a cognitive deficit per se, motor skills are controlled by the brain and certainly can be affected by brain trauma. The severity of involvement varies from subtle decreases in reaction time to slowed finger-thumb apposition to paralysis. Thus, the type of classroom interventions will be dependent upon the level of severity. In some instances, just allowing the student greater time to complete a written assignment will be necessary, while other cases might require special placement, such as in a physically handicapped classroom.

Interventions for Motor Impairments:

1. Allow the student greater time to complete written assignments.

2. Allow the student to complete assignments via computers and typewriters for which adaptive devices are available.

3. Encourage the student to use a clipboard for paper placement.

4. Work with the occupational therapist to develop appropriate instruments, such as "built up" pencils, clay pencil holders, page turners, weights on the wrist to control random and uncontrolled motor movements, and book holders. Adaptive devices for activities of daily living, such as "reachers," can assist the student to become more independent within the classroom. For children in wheelchairs, allow them to spend part of the school day using a stand-up table. This can prevent contractures and poor circulation and helps to maintain desired postural positions.

5. Assist the student to use a tape recorder or provide written notes.

6. Since most students with motor impairments receive occupational and physical therapy, it is important for the teacher to consult with these therapists regarding client specific treatment plans and adaptive devices.

General Classroom Recommendations

Due to the variability between students who are brain injured and the numerous interventions they may require within the classroom, it is essential that the teacher remain open and flexible. Being creative in modifying and adapting materials and the environment to meet the needs of the student who is brain injured can go a long way. But above all keep in mind that the overall purpose of intervention is to assist the student to carry out assignments and tasks independently. These classroom successes can bring pleasure and a sense of accomplishment to the brain injured student.

The following are suggestions of general classroom strategies to be used with the student who is brain injured:

1. Repetition and consistency are the keys to learning for the student who is brain injured.

2. Keep the environment free from distractors as much as possible.

3. Use concrete rather than abstract terms, familiar rather than novel material, and simple rather than complex directions.

4. Use tangible objects instead of numbers in teaching arithmetic.

5. Give clear, precise, short directions.

6. Check the student's level of understanding and interpretation of instructions and assignments.

7. Give shorter assignments.

8. Frequently review "new learning."

9. Provide one set of instructions at a time and avoid multi-step directions.

10. Present instructions and information both orally and with pictures.

11. Dramatize the information to be learned whenever possible.

12. Assist the student to make associations.

13. Use plenty of examples.

14. Use reinforcement to accelerate the learning process.

15. Use programmed instruction. Present material in small, logical steps, requiring the student to respond at each step. Give the student feedback regarding an answer before going on to the next step. This method of learning and computer assisted learning are very close in technique. They both allow students to proceed at their own rates.

16. Encourage and train the parents when possible to serve as "surrogate teachers" to facilitate generalization of learning.

17. Provide frequent, consistent breaks and/or vary complexity of classroom activities.

18. Provide the student with a brain injury with praise and encouragement.

19. Provide longer time limits for the brain injured child.

20. Be flexible and creative. Modify the curriculum if necessary.

21. Recommend tutorial services and educational remediation if necessary.

VI. ACADEMIC NEEDS AND STRATEGIES

The needs and strategies of students who are brain injured are closely tied to cognitive processing, since many of their learning problems are not premorbid learning disabilities but are the result of their cognitive deficits. There are similarities in the learning difficulties of individuals who are brain injured and learning disabled. However, the students with brain injury may have premorbid academic strengths and achievements and a strong motivation to return to that level; thus the hierarchical or "bottom-up" teaching, while necessary for the learning disabled, is inefficient for the student who is brain injured. While that student may exhibit global intellectual functioning similar to the mentally retarded, he can often reacquire a variety of premorbid skills and knowledge through the process of rehabilitation and educational re-entry, and frequently at a very fast rate. With the existing criteria for special services within the school system, many students who are brain injured do not qualify for these services. Thus, all teachers are presented with the need for additional information, skills, strategies, and materials for working with this population. Once the teacher understands the learning needs and patterns of these children through use of diagnostic information, observation, and daily measurement, educational programs can be implemented that use much of the knowledge, skills and materials already in the teacher's possession.

Before discussing specific academic needs and strategies, it may be helpful to reiterate some general principles for remediation which can be applied to the brain injured:

1. Individualize the problem.

2. Teach to the lowest level of involvement.

3. Teach to the type of involvement.

4. Teach according to readiness.

5. Remember that input precedes output.

6. Consider tolerance levels.

7. Consider the multisensory approach.

8. Remember to also teach to strengths, since teaching to deficits alone is limited.

9. Do not assume need for perceptual training.

10. Control important variables.

11. Emphasize both verbal and nonverbal learning.

Reading

Reading difficulties ultimately affect any student's performance in every academic subject area. While word recognition, spelling and comprehension are the most obvious and significant reading difficulties, the brain injured student's various cognitive deficiencies have an additional impact on reading competencies. The intent of reading remediation is to strengthen the weak or slow abilities or, as is often the case with the student who is brain injured, substitute whole or more functional skills for the deficient or impaired ones. There are many cognitive functions involved in the act of reading, including sensori-motor skills, visual perceptual skills, and auditory perception. In teaching or retraining it is not always possible or necessary to separate the functions, since one remedial strategy may impact several functions simultaneously.

Diagnostic information should make the distinction between visual and auditory reading disorders, as well as a variety of comprehension difficulties. Those students experiencing visual difficulties may exhibit confusion of similar letters and words, frequent letter reversals and inversions, and poor visual sequencing, visual memory, visual analysis and visual integration skills. On the other hand, those with auditory reading disorders have difficulty blending sounds, reauditorizing phonemes and words, and learning phonetic word skills in general. Simultaneous integration of reading, writing and spelling is helpful, with an extended period of readiness training, before attempting to employ phonetic methods.

SCIENCE USED TO BE MY FAVORITE SUBJECT, BUT I DON'T UNDERSTAND THIS JUNK ANYMORE.

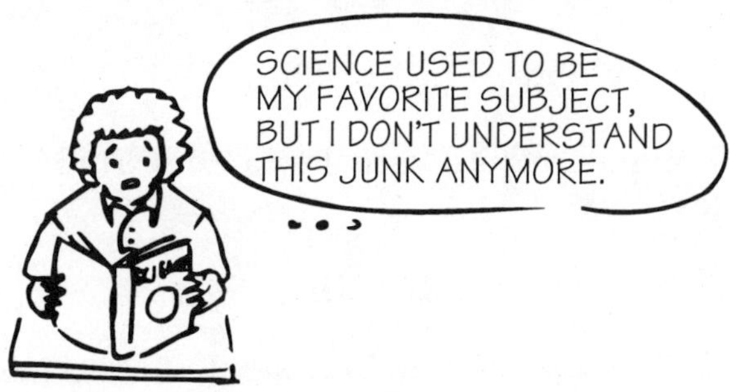

With age, higher thought processes become more significant in the reading process. It becomes more important to be able to keep a thought in mind for a longer period of time, and to manipulate ideas and develop mental abilities which lead to comprehension and judgment of the written words in terms of concept formation, manipulation of relationships, translation of symbols and other higher cognitive functions.

The student who is brain injured may experience a variety of reading difficulties. Just as any or all of the problems can be found in any age students with brain injury, depending on the location and severity of the injury, the suggestions for remedial activities and/or materials may be adapted to the appropriate age or ability level.

Remediation of word recognition and spelling difficulties (dysgraphia) is most effective when using the multimodal approach through auditory, visual and kinesthetic channels. Have the student repeat a word which has been presented orally, trace or copy the written word, find the word among several, and complete the word by filling in missing elements. Spelling rules may be of little or no help to those with memory problems, since they must be remembered in order to be used effectively. For those with memory difficulties, requiring the student to restate, either orally or in writing in his or her own words (encoding), the materials read serves the dual purpose of providing repetition and a measure of comprehension to both the student and the teacher. When decoding skills are inadequate, content needs to be adapted and work should be untimed.

For those with auditory perception problems, a visual whole-word or kinesthetic approach can be helpful. Even children who show no significant deficits in either auditory or visual processing can still experience difficulty with the association of auditory and visual stimuli. Methods such as VAKT (visual, auditory, kinesthetic and tactile) can be used to help associate these two sensory channels. For example, the child is told to jump while reading the word jump. For those with auditory deficits and problems retaining sequencing of sounds, listening skills training and use of picture cards can help with word recognition, rather than using the phonics method too early.

Word recognition skills can be improved by having the student use a word in context, then presenting the same word in a new context and referring back to the student's own previous use of the word. Follow with word, phrase or sentence matching devices. This helps with both basic recognition and carryover.

For those with visual perceptual difficulties, such as visual analysis or visual synthesis of words, auditory skills should be emphasized through phonics workbooks and linguistic readers. This will help the student recognize the connection between the auditory stimulus and the actual letters and words, as well as the sounds of individual letters and common letter combinations. Use of a marker, ruler or trailing pencil may compensate for defective eye movements and improve reading skills.

Use of audiotapes, a reader or study buddy are helpful to those with visual perceptual difficulties. Reading orally contributes toward strengthening the relationship between the auditory and visual word and gives reinforcement of the content of the material. As speed increases, single word identification and word attack skills may return to premorbid levels before comprehension does.

Relating reading assignments and activities to the brain injured student's relevant prior knowledge increases comprehension, since this information may be more accessible than new, unfamiliar information. Linking new information in this way provides a way of remembering it more efficiently.

Math

Requisite to understanding and correctly using the decimal (base ten) system of numeration is the ability to group, match, sort, compare and relate. These are the building blocks with which more complex concepts, operations, and abstract reasoning are built. Errors can occur because of lack of understanding the concepts, lack of understanding the language and symbols used to express the concepts, or simple computational errors.

In dealing with mathematics and the student with a brain injury, it is important to remember again the several cognitive variables which may affect understanding and performance in this area: attention/concentration deficits, memory problems, perceptual deficits, and sequencing difficulties, as well as language and clerical difficulties. Diagnostic information distinguishes between math disorders which relate to reading comprehension problems and those related to disturbances in quantitative thinking. Remediation choices should take into account other difficulties the student with a brain injury may be experiencing. When choosing a technique or strategy for remedial use, whether a child is a visual or auditory learner, or a sequential or simultaneous processor, must be considered. Again, the suggestions that follow may be adapted for the appropriate age or grade level.

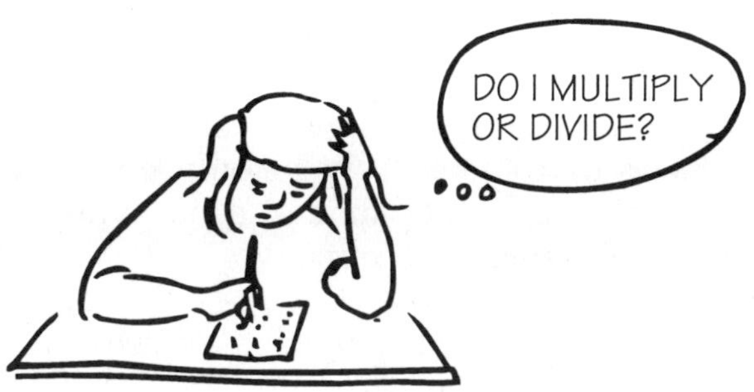

The student who is brain injured frequently thinks and speaks in concrete, literal terms, making abstract number concepts and operations difficult. For concrete demonstration of numbers and number manipulation, use of an abacus or real items can help to illustrate and translate numbers and operations into reality. Use of pictures and word problems which relate personally in some way to the student employ a multisensory approach to the concept. These also demonstrate the use of concepts and operations in a variety of contexts, as well as the use of such factors as fractions, time, weight, and temperature.

Sequencing difficulties create a variety of problems in math. At the lowest level, a multimodal approach is best - listening, verbalizing, tracing, reading, and recalling a sequence of numbers and operational steps, such as in borrowing, carrying, multiplication and division. For those who cannot recall the steps of a process, a sample problem can be given as a model. To increase structure, the steps may be numbered or in different colors for cuing. Computer-directed and computer-enhanced instruction can also be used effectively to provide maximum structure and feedback for sequencing difficulties.

Memory deficits can affect recall of basic math language, concepts and computations. It may be necessary to start with cards which progressively match numbers and items by color, numbers with number of items, symbols and names, and symbols and numbers, and which move on to operational and conceptual work only after repeated exposure and review through consistent drill work. Since basic math facts rely heavily on memorization, use of calculators makes sense and reduces frustration for some students.

Visual-perceptual deficits may require visual cues to be given, indicating how the mathematical material is to be read, i.e., whether from left to right or top to bottom. Lining up columns of numbers correctly, keeping the decimal point in the proper position, and subtracting downward may avoid computational errors which are, in fact, due to visual perceptual difficulties. Use of graph paper for orientation and use of association to recall direction of operation ("subtract means go down like a submarine" or "make sure things add up") should prove helpful. Use of puzzles, pegboards, and three dimensional shapes will help in the area of spatial perception and recognizing part to whole relationships.

Whenever possible, concrete, manipulative materials should be employed. Through use of these materials and minute sequential steps carefully paced and used in conjunction with word problems to help generalize each new factor or concept learned, progress can be made.

Language

Language is the means by which we communicate through both the written and spoken word. Language is important in forming and shaping thought, a very basic requirement for pragmatics, social interaction, abstract thinking and reasoning, and academics. These language and communication skills are often affected by brain injury. Many are serious enough to qualify for the special services of a speech clinician. There are often children who have suffered a brain injury and appear to have adequate expressive and written language skills. In reality, however, they may experience a variety of subtle language deficiencies which may cause difficulty in a number of areas. These children generally express themselves in concrete terms, are very rigid in concept formation, have difficulty generalizing and categorizing, and tend toward abnormal abstraction or generalization.

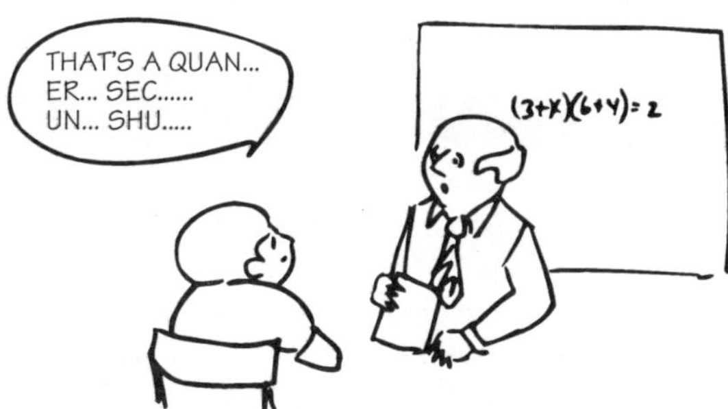

Other expressive language difficulties which are frequently seen following brain trauma are decreased verbal fluency, word finding difficulties, improper syntax, impaired visual naming, impaired auditory comprehension, and associated reading and writing problems. Those with impaired expressive language skills may display difficulty in initiating conversations or answering questions which require forming thoughts and/or drawing conclusions. This affects pragmatics and, ultimately, social relationships when these children experience difficulty communicating in group and social situations. They often may attempt to control situations, respond inappropriately to others' feelings, have difficulty initiating or taking part in conversation, or use abnormally fast or slow speech. The language of children with brain injuries often consists of limited vocabularies, circumlocutions, semantic approximations, and concrete representations, and they may use behavior as a means of communication.

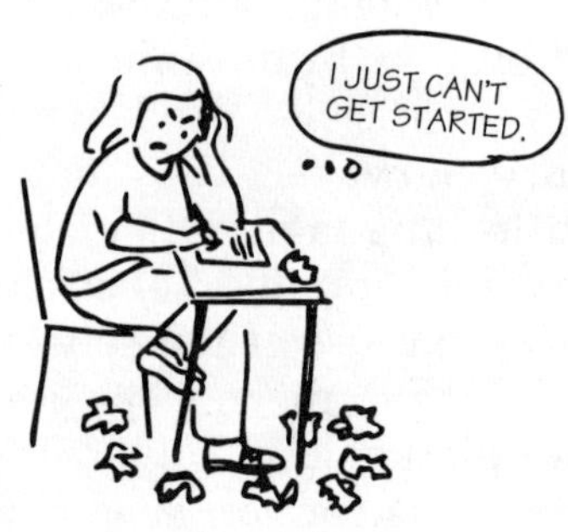

Written language can be affected by visual and auditory processing deficits. Students may not recognize spelling mistakes in words which they understand when orally presented. They may exhibit limited vocabulary in written work, often with inappropriate words or words out of context, and they may write just what is heard or demonstrate difficulty sequencing or comprehending directions or reading material. Those with auditory processing or language comprehension problems may have trouble understanding speech that is rapid or complex and, consequently, guess or pretend to understand. Frequently these children will ultimately avoid the spoken exchange and/or written assignments because of these difficulties and the resulting frustration.

To help these students, classroom activities should be developed which not only support clinicians' therapies, but which also provide exposure, encouragement, involvement, interest, variety, opportunity, and innovation in order to maximize speech and language usage. Instructions and assignments should be given as simply and clearly as possible. Again, using both oral and written modes will help connect the two. Use concrete language and limit the amount of information given. Demonstrate or act out directions. Ask students to repeat what they hear - verbal rehearsal - once, and then again using different words. To provide a variety of language experiences, tapes, stories, games and film strips with subtitles may be used. Encourage oral reading. Require that answers be given in complete, grammatically correct sentences, both orally and written. Pair verbal information with pictures or signs. Use cue cards, pictorial or written, to go with directions or instructions. For problems with pragmatics, the use of prompting, modelling, acting out or role-playing to increase appropriateness and sensitivity to others or the situation.

In addition to individualized instruction within the academic environment, a variety of other modifications may be implemented that increase the effectiveness of teaching the student with a brain injury, such as:

1. Ability grouping.

2. A shortened school day.

3. Frequent rest periods.

4. Modification of materials.

5. Use of compensatory equipment (calculator, tape recorder, typewriter, etc.).

6. Additional processing or work time.

7. Assignments given both verbally and in written form.

8. Shorter assignments.

9. Testing modifications such as oral, open book or take home.

10. Schedule and task guides.

11. Assignment/accomplishment notebook.

12. Tutoring and/or a study buddy.

13. Teaching good study skills such as the PQ4R method.

Teaching the student who is brain injured does not end in the classroom. Parents need to become familiar with the approach being used in school so that they can review and reinforce at home, thus providing consistent opportunities for academic development or retraining. Teachers and parents working as a team should be applying meaningful support and help, with the ultimate goal of helping these students to direct their own behaviors appropriately.

VII. EVALUATION INSTRUMENTS AND CONSIDERATIONS

An essential part of the process of teaching a student with a brain injury is an accurate evaluation and diagnosis of the student's injury, residual effects, and current strengths and weaknesses in physical, cognitive, and behavioral/emotional domains. As each child and their particular constellation of functional deficits is unique, it is of vital importance that you, as an educator, have a working knowledge of the evaluation instruments used to determine the child's needs. Generally, medical and psychological test results will need to be interpreted by trained professionals in their respective fields. A wide variety of cognitive and academic measures are also used in evaluating students who are brain injured, and they can provide you with a good working knowledge of your students' strengths and weaknesses. If you are familiar with these test instruments and what they purport to measure, you will be able to use the test results appropriately in determining instructional methods and strategies. Keep in mind, however, that specific test results are influenced by a wide variety of factors. Conclusions or interpretations should be made with caution. As the teacher, you can and should draw upon the knowledge and experience of professionals in each area of evaluation to aid you in reaching the most appropriate conclusions and developing appropriate instructional programs.

You may already be familiar with many of the more popular diagnostic instruments used to assess intellectual functioning, learning disabilities, and academic functioning. In evaluating students with brain injury, many of the same instruments are used, along with other neuropsychological tests. Interpretation, however, of specific test results may be different than for a learning disabled or developmentally delayed student who does not have a brain injury, as the nature of the injury typically has quite specific consequences.

First, with most mild to moderate closed head injuries, old learning is often relatively unaffected. The student's ability to attend and learn new information, however, may be significantly compromised. Thus, intellectual scores on a standard IQ test (such as the WISC-R or WAIS-R) may be close or equal to premorbid levels, as these tests generally measure old learning. One cannot assume, however, that average IQ scores mean the student has a normal ability to learn new information. Making such an assumption would be overestimating the child's abilities, resulting in much frustration, both for the student and for you as a teacher.

Secondly, although a student who is brain injured may be able to perform relatively distinct tasks in a structured test setting, one cannot assume that those skills will be transferable to a classroom or real life setting. Many students who are brain injured have significant difficulties with initiation, planning, organization, perception, and integration of information. Thus, even mild deficits noted in testing may reflect significant functional deficits and should be taken seriously.

A third common residual effect of brain injury is an overall decrease in cognitive processing speed. This may be reflected in a decreased performance IQ on the WISC-R or WAIS-R, due to the timed nature of tasks, or on other tests where speed of processing is relevant. Low scores on such test instruments should not be interpreted to mean the student cannot understand or complete the task; rather, they may not be able to do so in a timely manner or under pressure. Given adequate time to process and respond, however, they may often be able to perform many more tasks than originally assumed or indicated by test scores.

The child's age at time of injury is also a significant factor in terms of test interpretation and prognosis. It was once generally assumed that the younger the age at injury, the greater the prognosis for recovery. This was based on the belief that the brain's general elasticity and capacity at a younger age permits it to modify itself to compensate for damaged components. It is becoming increasingly evident, however, that even mild brain injuries at younger ages may have far-reaching and significant effects in the child's ultimate overall level of functioning. This is undoubtedly due in large part to the effects on attention, memory, and learning of new information. Older children, having already learned more basic skills and information, generally retain these skills or can relearn old skills more quickly. Younger children have a more limited base of "old learning," and must struggle to a greater degree to attain even basic skills. In addition, the normal variability in functioning expected at younger ages adds to the complexity of interpreting test results at these ages.

In light of all of these factors, the making of strong prognostic statements relative to the potential functioning of very young students who are brain injured based on specific test results needs to be done with the utmost caution and only in the most conservative manner. Frequent reevaluation and charting of progress as the child grows and learns will be necessary in order to make useful inferences and as accurate a prognosis as possible.

In this chapter, we will review several widely used cognitive and academic test instruments in order to familiarize you with their names and purposes. The list is, of course, not exhaustive. There are many excellent diagnostic tools in use in school systems, hospitals, and rehabilitative centers. The instruments covered here, however, are currently some of the most frequently used and accepted for diagnostic and placement purposes in the school districts.

Cognitive Processing Instruments

Woodcock-Johnson PsychoEducational Battery -Revised

This instrument purports to measure seven cognitive factors, as well as four areas of scholastic aptitude. The following outline lists each of the seven cognitive factors and the subtests comprising them.

1. Long-term Retrieval
   a. Memory for Names
   b. Visual Auditory Learning
   c. Delayed Recall

2. Short-term Memory
   a. Memory for Sentences
   b. Memory for Words
   c. Numbers Reversed

3. Processing Speed
   a. Visual Matching
   b. Cross Out

4. Auditory Processing
   a. Incomplete Words
   b. Sound Blending
   c. Sound Patterns

5. Visual Processing
   a. Visual Closure
   b. Picture Recognition
   c. Spatial Relations

6. Comprehension-Knowledge
   a. Picture Vocabulary

   b. Oral Vocabulary
   c. Listening Comprehension
   d. Verbal Analogies

7. Fluid Reasoning
   a. Analysis-Synthesis
   b. Concept Formation
   c. Spatial Relations
   d. Verbal Analysis

Detroit Test of Learning Aptitude - 2

The DTLA-2 is comprised of 11 subtests which form nine composite scores representing four general domains. These domains, composites, and the subtests comprising them are listed below. In addition, the Total Test score is comprised of all subtests.

1. Linguistic Domain
   a. Verbal Aptitude Composite
      1) Word Opposites
      2) Sentence Imitation
      3) Oral Directions
      4) Word Sequences
      5) Story Construction
      6) Word Fragments
   b. Nonverbal Aptitude Composite
      1) Design Reproduction
      2) Object Sequences
      3) Symbolic Relations
      4) Conceptual Matching
      5) Letter Sequences

2. Cognitive Domain
   a. Conceptual Aptitude Composite
      1) Word Opposites
      2) Sentence Imitation
      3) Oral Directions
      4) Story Construction
      5) Symbolic Relations
      6) Conceptual Matching

7) Word Fragments

b. Structural Aptitude Composite
   1) Word Sequences
   2) Design Reproductions
   3) Object Sequences
   4) Letter Sequences

3. Attentional Domain
   a. Attention Enhanced Aptitude Composite
      1) Sentence Imitation
      2) Oral Directions
      3) Word Sequences
      4) Design Reproduction
      5) Object Sequences
      6) Letter Sequences
   b. Attention Reduced Aptitude Composite
      1) Word Opposites
      2) Story Construction
      3) Symbolic Relations
      4) Conceptual Matching
      5) Word Fragments

4. Motoric Domain
   a. Motor Enhanced Aptitude Composite
      1) Oral Directions
      2) Design Reproduction
      3) Object Sequences
      4) Letter Sequences
   b. Motor Reduced Aptitude Composite
      1) Word Opposites
      2) Sentence Imitation
      3) Word Sequences
      4) Story Construction
      5) Symbolic Relations
      6) Conceptual Matching
      7) Word Fragments

Kaufman - Assessment Battery for Children

The K-ABC is comprised of ten cognitive processing subtests, resulting in two composite scales and an overall composite score. This test is based on the sequential/simultaneous approach discussed in a previous chapter.

1. Sequential Processing
    a. Hand Movements
    b. Number Recall
    c. Word Order

2. Simultaneous Processing
    a. Magic Window
    b. Face Recognition
    c. Gestalt Closure
    d. Triangles
    e. Matrix Analogies
    f. Spatial Memory
    g. Photo Series

Other Cognitive Processing Tests

In addition to the three listed above, you may see other cognitive processing instruments frequently used. These may include the Illinois Test of Psycholinguistic Abilities (ITPA), Bender Visual Motor Gestalt Test, and Beery Test of Visual Motor Integration just to name a few. Again, although it is generally recommended that specific tests be interpreted by professionals trained in the area of assessment relative to those specific tests, it will be helpful for you to be familiar with the names and general nature of these instruments in order to aid your students.

Academic Test Instruments

Woodcock-Johnson PsychoEducational Battery -Revised

This instrument measures achievement in three broad areas of reading, mathematics, and written language, as well as general knowledge and special skills.

1. Reading
    a. Broad Reading
        1) Letter-Word Identification
        2) Passage Comprehension
    b. Basic Reading Skills
        1) Letter-Word Identification
        2) Word Attack
    c. Reading Comprehension
        1) Passage Comprehension
        2) Reading Vocabulary

2. Mathematics
    a. Broad Mathematics
        1) Calculation
        2) Applied Problems
    b. Basic Skills
        1) Calculation
        2) Quantitative Concepts
    c. Reasoning
        1) Applied Problems
    d. Broad Mathematics
        1) Calculation
        2) Applied Problems
    e. Basic Skills
        1) Calculation
        2) Quantitative Concepts
    f. Reasoning
        1) Applied Problems

3. Written Language
    a. Broad Written Language
        1) Dictation
        2) Writing Samples
    b. Basic Skills
        1) Dictation
        2) Proofing
    c. Expression
        1) Writing Samples
        2) Writing Fluency
    d. Punctuation, Spelling, and Usage
        1) Dictation
        2) Proofing

e. Handwriting
    1) Writing Samples

4. Broad Knowledge Cluster
    a. Science
    b. Social Studies
    c. Humanities

5. Skills Cluster
    a. Letter-Word Identification
    b. Applied Problems
    c. Dictation

Wide Range Achievement Test - Revised

The WRAT-R is a widely used academic screening instrument which provides limited, but often useful, information relative to general skill levels in three areas. Due to the limited scope of this instrument, it is most appropriately used as a screening test, with more comprehensive achievement tests to be used for more specific diagnosis and remediation recommendations.

1. Reading (recognition)

2. Spelling

3. Arithmetic (computation)

Kaufman - Test of Educational Achievement

The K-TEA measures three general areas of reading, mathematics, and spelling.

1. Reading Area
    a. Reading Decoding
    b. Reading Comprehension

2. Mathematics
    a. Mathematics Applications
    b. Mathematics Computation

3. Spelling

Peabody Individual Achievement Test - Revised

The PIAT-R is comprised of five subtests, and results in composite scores for Reading and the Total Test. Written Expression is measured separately.

1. Reading
   a. General Information
   b. Reading Recognition
   c. Reading Comprehension

2. Mathematics

3. Spelling

4. Written Expression

Kaufman-Assessment Battery for Children

In addition to the cognitive processing scales, the K-ABC also includes an achievement battery. The scale results in six individual subtest scores and one overall achievement score that is then compared to cognitive processing scales.

1. Expressive vocabulary

2. Faces and places

3. Arithmetic

4. Riddles

5. Reading/decoding

6. Reading/understanding

Relating Test Scores/Instruments to Cognitive Processing Areas

As you can see, each instrument has its own organization and grouping of particular tests to measure specific cognitive processes and academic skills. In order to aid you in more easily determining the cognitive area tapped by certain tests, the following charts are offered. So you can easily refer to strategies recommended in Chapter 5 relative to each area.

WOODCOCK-JOHNSON PSYCHOEDUCATIONAL BATTERY

	Attention / Concentration	Auditory Memory	Visual Memory	Sequencing	Auditory Comprehension	Visual Comprehension	Problem Solving	Organization	Motor	Processing Speed
1. Memory for Name	X	X	X							
2. Memory for Sentence	X	X		X						
3. Visual Matching	X								X	X
4. Incomplete Words	X				X					
5. Visual Closure						X				
6. Picture Vocabulary						X				
7. Analysis-Synthesis	X						X			
8. Visual-Auditory Learning	X	X	X							
9. Memory for Words	X	X								
10. Cross Out	X								X	X
11. Sound Blending	X				X					
12. Picture Recognition						X				
13. Oral Vocabulary					X					
14. Concept Formation	X						X			
15. Delayed Memory for Names		X								
16. Delayed Vis-Aud Learning		X	X							
17. Numbers Reversed	X	X								
18. Sound Patterns	X				X					
19. Spatial Relations	X					X				
20. Listening Comprehension	X				X					
21. Verbal Analogies					X					

DETROIT TESTS OF LEARNING APTITUDE-2

	Attention / Concentration	Auditory Memory	Visual Memory	Sequencing	Auditory Comprehension	Visual Comprehension	Problem Solving	Organization	Motor	Processing Speed
1. Word Opposites					X					
2. Sentence Imitation	X	X		X						
3. Oral Directions	X	X			X	X			X	
4. Word Sequences	X	X								
5. Story Construction				X	X			X		
6. Design Reproduction	X		X			X			X	
7. Object Sequences	X		X						X	
8. Symbolic Relations						X	X			
9. Conceptual Matching						X				
10. Word Fragments						X				
11. Letter Sequences	X	X								

KAUFMAN-ASSESSMENT BATTERY FOR CHILDREN (COGNITIVE)

	Attention / Concentration	Auditory Memory	Visual Memory	Sequencing	Auditory Comprehension	Visual Comprehension	Problem Solving	Organization	Motor	Processing Speed
1. Magic Window	X					X				
2. Face Recognition	X		X			X		X		
3. Hand Movement	X		X	X				X	X	
4. Gestalt Closure						X				
5. Number Recall	X	X		X						
6. Triangles						X	X	X	X	X
7. Word Order	X	X		X	X	X				
8. Matrix Analogies						X	X	X		
9. Spatial Memory	X		X			X		X		
10. Photo Series	X			X		X	X	X		

VIII. BEHAVIORAL NEEDS AND STRATEGIES

One of the most common barriers to the successful educational re-entry of children who are brain injured is the development of classroom behavior problems. These behaviors can range from subtle to quite disruptive. The most common behavior problems associated with brain injury are listed below. Although many of these behaviors often occur in any classroom, the frequency and/or intensity is often much greater in the child who has sustained a brain injury.

In this section, we will not only attempt to identify common behavior problems, but also offer a practical strategy and specific techniques for the classroom management of these behaviors. The general strategy presented here is called behavior analysis, and is supported by over 40 years of research. Behavior analysis has been demonstrated as an effective method for understanding and, ultimately, changing the maladaptive behaviors associated with traumatic brain injury. The hallmark of behavior analysis is the identification of the variable or variables maintaining the target behavior. In other words, the first task of behavior change is to identify the current source (or sources) of motivation for the problem behavior. Once we know why a behavior occurs, we can often change it by removing the source of motivation for the undesired behavior and providing a more desirable one.

The following examples illustrate how a behavioral analysis can be used in the classroom to address some common behaviors displayed by children who are brain injured.

Disruptiveness

Children who are brain injured are often described as impulsive because of their high activity and attention-getting behaviors. In the classroom, the most common disruptive behaviors include physical aggression, speaking out of turn, refusing to stay seated, and teasing or taunting of others.

Examples:

1. The teacher asks a hypothetical question and the student yells out an answer.

2. During a silent reading period, the student loudly taps a pencil on the desk.

3. A student answers incorrectly, and the student who is brain injured publicly berates the student for the mistake.

Classroom Interventions for Disruptiveness:

The above behaviors could be motivated by many sources. The most common is attention. Generally, a common denominator of all disruptive behaviors is a focusing of attention upon the disruptive individual. This attention may be positive (smiles or snickers from peers) or negative (teacher and/or student reprimands).

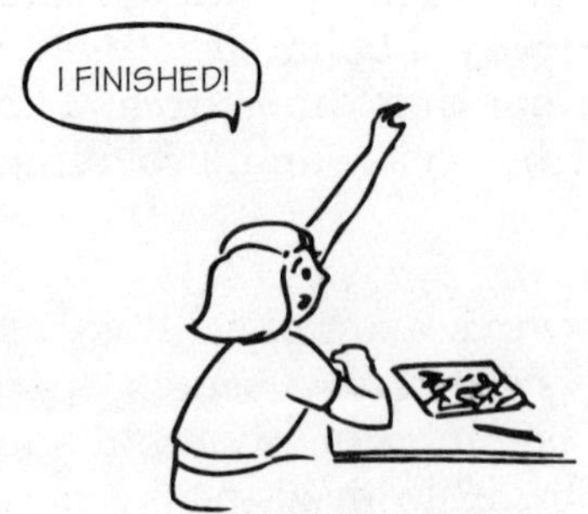

In the child who is brain injured, attention, either positive or negative, may be a very positive motivator of behavior. One explanation for this propensity for engaging in disruptive, attention-getting behaviors is the injured student's reduced repertoire of behaviors. That is, the child who is brain injured may have more difficulty obtaining attention from others in appropriate ways (e.g., performing well in school, being popular with peers) due to the cognitive and/or social skills deficits as a result of the accident. Since disruptive behaviors are generally a reliable method of obtaining attention in the classroom, the student who is brain injured is particularly likely to engage in these behaviors.

To decrease attention-motivated disruptiveness, the teacher must eliminate attention (both positive and negative) for disruptive behaviors, and provide attention for appropriate classroom behaviors. The most direct technique for managing attention-motivated disruptive behavior is to lavish the disruptive student with attention when appropriate behavior is displayed. If attention is sought, provide it liberally for the absence of disruption. That is, make an effort to catch a disruptive child being good. If the classroom is too large or the frequency of attention necessary too great for the teacher to manage, perhaps a teacher's aide or assistant could be assigned the task of catching the disruptive child being good.

We find that the use of frequent attention for appropriate behavior, in combination with the absence of attention for disruptive behavior, can produce immediate and dramatic results.

Noncompliance

For our purposes, noncompliance is defined as refusal to follow the teacher's requests. In addition to this being quite disruptive in the classroom, noncompliance also has important implications for basic student-teacher relationships. It has been repeatedly demonstrated that an increase in student compliance often results in an improvement in many, non-targeted classroom behaviors (e.g., disruptive behaviors). Common examples of classroom noncompliance are listed below.

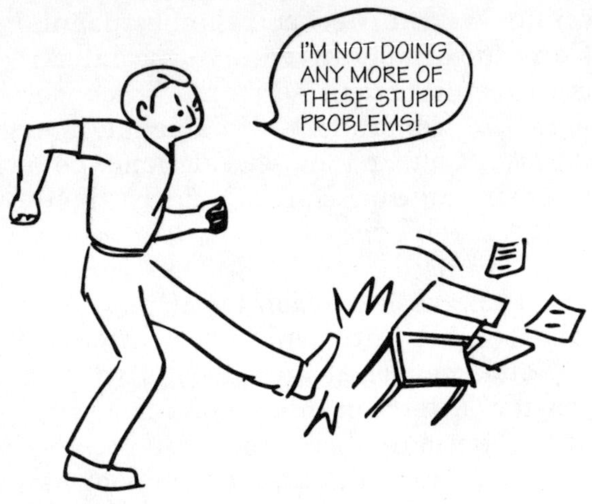

Examples:

1. The student who is brain injured continues talking to classmates, despite several requests to stop.

2. In response to the teacher's requests to "not" open a book, the noncompliant student immediately opens the book.

3. The student refuses to answer a question, even though the answer is known.

Classroom Interventions for Noncompliance:

Noncompliance can be maintained by several sources of motivation. As in disruptive behaviors, noncompliance may occur in response to the brain injured child's attempts to regain attention from the environment. If the noncompliance is primarily motivated by teacher or peer attention, then a strategy as outlined above (for disruptive behaviors) would be an effective intervention to establish compliance. Specifically, in attention-motivated students, the teacher would provide attention for compliant behavior and eliminate attention for noncompliance. The teacher may "stack the deck" by initially asking noncompliant students to do things they are likely to want to do. Of course, the most critical component when dealing with the attention-motivated student is that they learn that much more attention is provided for compliance rather than noncompliance.

Noncompliance may also be motivated by other sources. A child may be noncompliant in order to escape or avoid school or teacher requests. Dealing with the noncompliant student can be so aversive that teachers may unintentionally avoid the student. Students who are brain injured may be motivated by this escape or avoidance of teacher demands because school has become unpleasant. The difficulty that many children with brain injury have with school may be caused by several reasons (e.g., cognitive deficits, missed school, fatigue, poor relationships with peers), but noncompliance and uncooperativeness may serve as an effective way to minimize teacher/academic demands.

The classroom intervention for escape-motivated noncompliance is a twofold approach. First, it is important to reestablish school as a pleasant activity. This may be accomplished by modifying the brain injured student's curriculum and academic demands to maximize opportunities for success. Secondly, make a conscious effort to insure that the student does not escape or avoid academic opportunities or challenges due to noncompliance or uncooperativeness.

Lack of Initiation/Motivation

Heretofore we have been discussing classroom behavior problems commonly associated with increased activity following a brain injury. However, one of the biggest challenges to teachers is the motivation of the unresponsive students.

Examples:

1. The students appear to be lethargic, showing little or no interest in activities the other students enjoy.

2. When asked what they would like to do, the students shrug their shoulders and stare off blankly.

3. The students' classwork is slow, and assignments are seldom completed.

Classroom Intervention for Lack of Initiation and Motivation:

Lack of initiation and a flat affect are common phenomena following a brain injury. Recently injured students may be confused and fatigued due to the insult to the brain and the effects of medications. The extent of recovery and the time of this process is individualized, and, unfortunately, impossible to accurately predict. However, if you have a recovering brain injured student in your class, there are several things you can do to foster the child's readjustment to school. First, speak to the student's parents and physician, if possible, to identify the student's current medical, physical, and psychological status. Initially, a modification of curriculum may be necessary, which can gradually change from a part to a full school day.

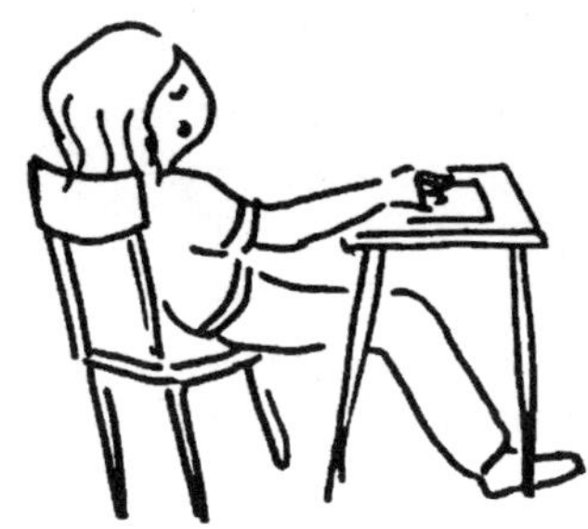

Additionally, a lack of initiation and motivation could be a learned behavior. Following a brain injury, an individual often becomes depressed because many of the things done prior to injury can no longer be done. Consequently, many of the things that were enjoyable and motivating, such as sports or school, are now difficult and have lost their ability to motivate. Accordingly, the student who is brain injured learns that no matter what, access to those things that are most enjoyable to him cannot be accomplished. As a result of this condition, the brain injured student stops responding.

The most effective strategy for these children is to try to establish new, obtainable goals and enjoyable activities. Asking unresponsive brain injured students what they like may not prove fruitful, but arranging for the students to sample novel activities may be a valuable way of identifying some new motivators. The important point is to understand that the students may lack initiation because they have learned that their efforts no longer get them what they want. The solution then is to help these students identify realistic goals and new, enjoyable activities, and show them that these goals can be attained through their own efforts.

In summary, all of the management techniques discussed above are familiar to most classroom teachers. Our emphasis in this section is that these commonly used techniques are most effectively applied when the teacher understands why the undesirable behavior occurs.

All of the examples presented here assume the most common motivations, and assume behaviors that are maintained by only one source of motivation. Of course, some behaviors may be affected by several variables and, therefore, require a combination of interventions. Additionally, some behaviors such as severe physical aggression and self-injurious behavior will require consultation with experts in brain injury. However, it is our experience that the use of these strategies can aid the teacher in successfully managing the behavior of a student who is brain injured.

IX. TEACHER REACTIONS TO TEACHING STUDENTS WITH BRAIN INJURY

As a teacher of a student who is brain injured, an awareness of the cognitive, academic, and behavioral needs is obviously important in enabling you to appropriately work with that individual. Equally important, however, is awareness of the fact that as the teacher you will also experience emotional and/or behavioral changes as a result of your interaction with that student. Your reactions will vary depending upon the nature and extent of the difficulties your student is experiencing. The more challenging the difficulty presented, the more likely you as the teacher will experience one or more of the negative reactions described in this section.

The first step in effectively handling your own reactions to teaching students who have brain injury is to gain knowledge and awareness of the most frequently experienced feelings. This awareness will prepare you to cope more effectively with feelings you may experience and reduce the tendency to blame yourself for problems which may arise.

The second step is recognition. In order to cope effectively, you must be able to recognize your own negative reactions, their nature and intensity, as they occur. You must be vigilant about monitoring your feelings and behavior by frequently asking yourself, "What feelings am I experiencing?" or "What am I thinking about this situation?" Observe your own body language, tone of voice, words, and actions. In doing so, you will learn to recognize the nature and intensity of your own reactions in teaching students with brain injury.

The third step is action. When you recognize negative reactions in yourself, you must take positive action to change them. The change could be in the nature of the reaction or a reduction of its intensity. By gaining an awareness of your own negative reactions, as well as the ability to recognize and change them, you will gain significant confidence, control, and competence in teaching the students with brain injury.

In this section, we will present several typical negative reactions and general strategies or guidelines for coping with them. Of course, this is not an exhaustive list, and suggestions would need to be tailored to each individual situation, as well as your own personal needs. As a professional educator, you are well equipped to adapt these suggestions to your personal situations, drawing upon your own experience and creativity to develop the most appropriate coping strategies.

Overoptimism/Unrealistic Expectations

"I just don't understand what the problem is. Johnny just isn't progressing the way he should."

One of the most common reactions to teaching students with brain injury, overoptimism, stems from a lack of knowledge or understanding of the results of a brain injury. Excessive demands are often made upon students as a result of the unrealistic expectations placed upon them by others. Unrealistic expectations are those that are not appropriate relative to the student's current functioning and future potential.

FOR TOMORROW DO PAGES
12-14 IN YOUR WORKBOOK,
FINISH READING CHAPTER 2,
WRITE 5 PARAGRAPHS ON...
WHA....

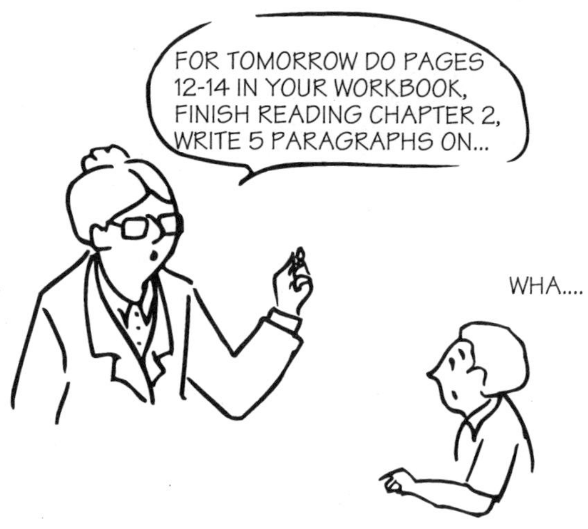

This lack of knowledge and understanding of what is realistic is common, as most teachers have little or no experience or frame of reference for dealing with individuals who are brain injured. You may not personally have ever known anyone with a brain injury prior to this point. Most individuals who sustained traumatic injuries prior to 10 to 15 years ago did not survive. Now, due to medical advances, individuals with serious injuries are surviving at a much greater rate and subsequently returning to the school setting. This creates a whole new group of students with special needs.

WHATTA THEY MEAN
"HEAD INJURED"?
HIS HEAD LOOKS
O.K. TO ME...

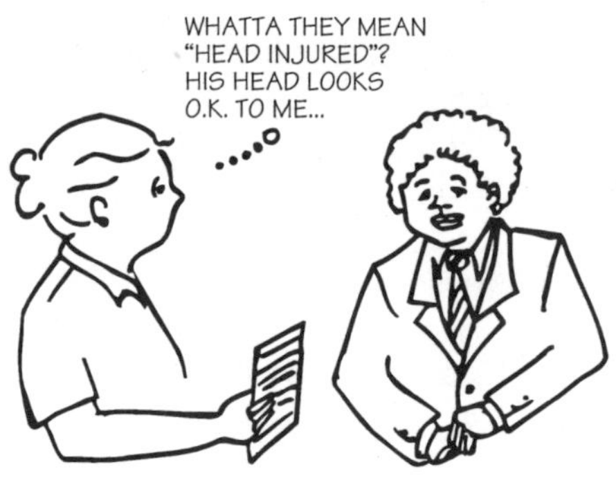

Another reason for unrealistic expectations or overoptimism is that the student often looks fine on the outside. That is, the injury or handicap is often not physically apparent, and the teacher may thus assume that there are no residual effects. Unlike with individuals who have an outer physical injury, such as a broken leg, there is often no immediate framework upon which to form appropriate expectations. Overoptimism may also stem from the teacher's overgeneralization from a few areas of high functioning. Students who are brain injured generally have some areas of ability that remain intact, and the teacher may wrongly assume that the student should be high functioning in all areas. This is known as the "halo" effect. And finally, you may have difficulty forming appropriate expectations relative to the brain injured student, because most teacher training programs do not include courses on brain injury. Thus, you may have little or no formal training on the neurobehavioral results of a brain injury. As a result, as a teacher you may lack both intuitive and formal knowledge that would aid in your understanding and ability to teach this population.

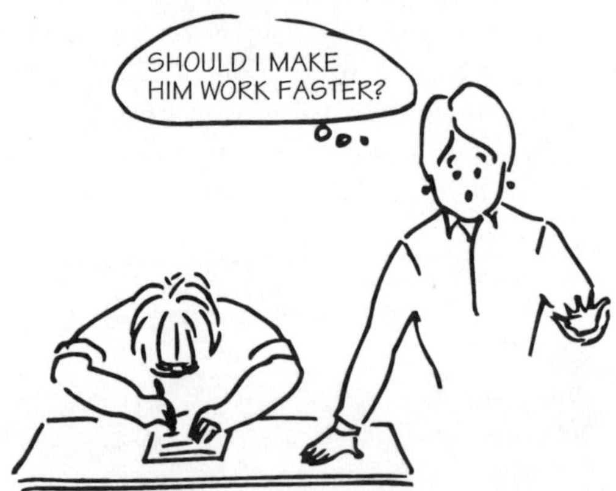

What feelings then result from this lack of knowledge? One of the most apparent and frequent is a general feeling of lack of self-confidence. As the student who is brain injured will inevitably experience more difficulty and failure than others, your self-esteem and feelings of competence will undoubtedly decrease if you assume that your student's lack of progress is a result of your own lack of ability to teach. You may experience feelings of helplessness, hopelessness, and eventually apathy. Frustration and anger may result, as well. As a professional educator, you certainly realize the impact of your expectations upon your student's learning and performance. Inappropriate expectations (either overly optimistic or pessimistic) can have a very negative effect upon your student's learning, as well as your own mental health. It is vitally important for you to become informed and develop a sense of competence and confidence in order to deal as effectively as possible with this population.

Strategies for Formulating Realistic Expectations

1. Gaining appropriate knowledge
   a. Read available information about the neurobehavioral results of brain injury. There are now many available articles, books, manuals, cassettes, videotapes, etc. with valuable and helpful information.
   b. Attend inservices and workshops on neuropsychology and brain injury.
   c. Study specific information regarding your individual students. Reports written by the team of professionals who worked with your students prior to returning to school will contain information regarding individual strengths, weaknesses, limitations, and needs.
   d. Consult directly with former therapists or professionals familiar with your students in order to gain more insight into their needs, limitations, and future potential.

2. Write down specific expectations for your student.
   a. Identify and rebut your initial unrealistic expectations using your new knowledge. Record

your unrealistic expectations on one half of a sheet of paper and rebut with the realistic expectation on the other half of the paper.

b. Monitor your own negative feelings. Recognize when you are experiencing a negative reaction and refer back to your list of expectations. Adjust expectations accordingly.

FRUSTRATION

"What's the use! I must have taught him that over a thousand times in a hundred different ways, and he still can't get it!"

One of the most common emotional reactions you may encounter in teaching the students with brain injury is frustration. This stems not only from lack of knowledge or unrealistic expectations, but from the fact that, even when armed with appropriate knowledge and seemingly realistic goals, the brain injured student will not always progress as you expect. There will be occasions when your goals are thwarted and expectations not achieved. Recall, if you will, the many cognitive, academic, and behavioral difficulties described in previous sections - attention and concentration deficits, memory deficits, inadequate judgment and reasoning, poor organization, lack of insight, impulsivity, irritability, immaturity, negative moods, and academic deficits, just to name a few. Even with extensive knowledge, the complexity of functional deficits results in frequent and unavoidable frustration for the teacher attempting to help this student.

Given the fact that you will encounter much frustration in teaching students with brain injury, what can you do to cope? First, you must realize and accept the idea that the student or situation itself is not causing your frustration. Frustration is an emotional reaction that you experience when your expectations are not achieved. Thus, it is important to accept your personal responsibility and control of your own frustration. Acceptance of this concept is important in managing frustration. It is not possible or desirable to totally avoid all frustration in your teaching of the students who are brain injured. Teachers who deny frustration lack insight, goals, or specific expectations for themselves or their students. There are, however, some general strategies which can be useful in helping you reduce the frequency and intensity of your feelings of frustration. As you gain better understanding of your own responsibility for your frustration, you will feel more confident and better equipped to help your students succeed.

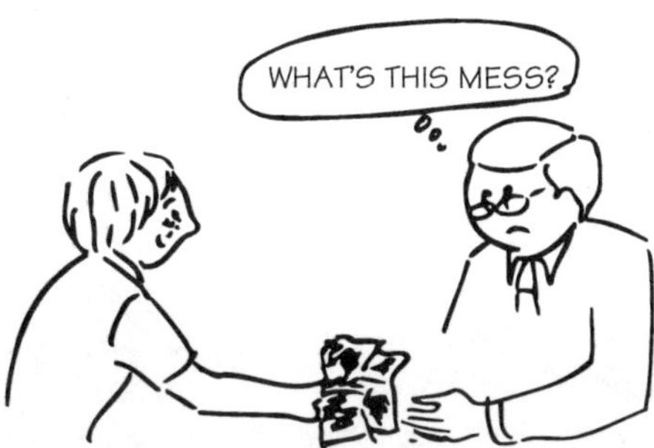

Strategies for Coping with Frustration

1. Recognize when you are feeling frustrated. Acknowledge these feelings of frustration to yourself. Accept these feelings as normal and expected. Remind yourself that frustration is your own reaction and not caused by the student or situation.

2. Identify which expectations are being thwarted, resulting in your frustration. Reassess the validity of these expectations. Are they realistic? (See previous section.) Adjust expectations to a more realistic level if appropriate.

3. Reexamine specific educational goals for your student. If overall expectations and primary goals appear to be appropriate and you continue to experience frustration, subgoals may need to be restructured or timelines for achieving goals adjusted in order to result in increased success. Adjust subgoals or timelines in a way that will provide increased success and decrease frustration for both yourself and your student.

4. Pinpoint the specific tasks that result in the most frustration for you or your student. Complete a task analysis of these tasks in order to identify the components resulting in frustration. Adjust educational strategies, taking into account your student's individual needs and the results of your task analysis.

5. Note those behaviors exhibited by your student that are most frustrating for you. Using your new knowledge and by consulting with professional support personnel, discriminate between those that can be changed or modified and those that cannot.
   a. Attempt to accept and adapt to those that cannot be changed, avoiding the tendency to interpret them as a personal affront or reflection on your own abilities. Recognize both your own and your student's limitations and adjust instructional activities accordingly.
   b. For those behaviors that you determine can be changed or modified, design and implement appropriate behavioral management strategies. Consult previous sections of this manual, as well as support personnel available to you, for specific ideas.

6. Participate in ongoing discussions with other teachers in similar situations. Seek opportunities to ventilate your frustrations to a sym-

pathetic ear in a positive and constructive atmosphere.

ANGER

"Jane - are you lazy, or just trying to make me mad? I've told you a thousand times to put your work in the basket when you're finished. You just don't listen!"

As frustration and disappointments build over time, you may eventually experience feelings of anger. Your student who is brain injured may appear to be not listening, not following directions, not caring, and generally not complying. With most students, both in regular and special education settings, such observations are indicative of attitude problems, learned negative behavior patterns, or manipulative behavior on the part of the student. These behaviors are then dealt with through a variety of disciplinary measures, both positive and negative. The critical factor here is willful and deliberate lack of compliance or manipulative behavior. In working with the brain injured, similar behavior patterns may need to be interpreted very differently. It is important to distinguish organic effects on behavior, personality, and learning from more common behavior disorders or manipulative tendencies. Remember the complexity of effects that can result from traumatic brain injury - it cannot and should not be assumed that a student who is brain injured can or will respond to learning or discipline in a "normal" way. Memory deficits are significant for many - routines and expectations may not be retained from day to day. Deficits in perception relate not only to cognitive tasks but to interpersonal interaction and communications, as well. The student may misread your intent, misinterpret directions, or draw inappropriate conclusions relative to behavioral expectations. Impulsivity reduces control over actions and responses - although a rule is known, the student with brain injury may act before thinking through the correct choices or behavior. Low motivation or lack of initiation may affect performance. These are just a few examples of possible direct residual effects of a brain injury (discussed in detail in previous sections) that may appear to be willful noncompliance or manipulative behavior to the uninformed eye. Recognizing these characteristics as expected effects, rather than attributing negative intent on the student's part, will help you reduce your anger toward the student or situation when they occur.

This is not to say that the student is not responsible for the behavior or should be "let off the hook." Rather, the way in which you as a teacher respond may need to be modified. A less punitive or disciplinary attitude or approach and a more positive and flexible approach may need to be taken. Previous sections have provided specific strategies for responding to certain behaviors and situations. As you begin to recognize these often aggravating characteristics as organically related, you will find yourself experiencing less anger toward your student.

There will be times, however, when you still feel anger. When anger does occur, it needs to be dealt with adaptively, rather than directed inwardly toward yourself or externally toward your student. In order to do so, you must begin to change how you interpret or think about events. It is not the student or event that makes us angry, but how we interpret or think about it that results in anger and determines the nature and intensity of the anger response.

Like frustration, anger is a negative emotion which can result in a hostile learning atmosphere if not controlled. There are several steps in controlling anger: first, awareness of your anger, its frequency and intensity; second, commitment to a strategy to deal with your anger and development of a plan of action; and third, follow-through on your plan. Many self-help books and extensive manuals have been written relative to dealing with anger. Become aware and discover those strategies that work best for you.

Strategies for Anger Control

1. Identify your expectations of your student. Eliminate the words "should," "ought," and "must" from your vocabulary. Evaluate your expectations and replace them as needed with realistic ones (see previous section).

2. List specific behaviors, situations and tasks that are sources of anger for you. Analyze these sources and change the teaching strategies, or environment to reduce anger provoking situations.

3. Be aware of your own level of stress. As your stress level increases, your frustration increases and anger control decreases. Seek information on stress reduction. Make sure you are taking care of yourself.

4. Seek information about anger control. For example:
   a. Identify irrational beliefs and mental distortions which contribute to anger. Substitute more rational thoughts.
   b. Use regulated breathing and relaxation techniques to aid control and reduce stress (e.g., counting to 10 before speaking, changing body position, speaking softly).

5. Keep your sense of humor. Avoid taking yourself too seriously. Laughter and humor can defuse many potentially anger laden situations.

6. Communicate your feelings assertively, not aggressively. Let the students know what you expect and have them help identify the problem and formulate solutions. As you communicate, you will become more aware of your students' perceptions and points of view and will find yourself becoming more empathetic and experiencing less anger.

We have reviewed in this section several typical reactions that teachers may experience in their teaching of students with brain injury. Your particular reactions may be similar, but may also include other negative feelings such as helplessness, guilt, or even apathy. It should be apparent at this time that the key to successful interaction with your brain injured students is knowledge - knowledge of both the students' characteristics and your own responses and reactions to your student. The challenge is great, but the rewards can be equally as great as you see the successes and progress that can be achieved with this population. Your ability to be flexible, adaptable, and tuned in to your students' needs will be of utmost importance.

X. PREPARING STUDENTS WITH BRAIN INJURY FOR VOCATIONS

Background and Problems

The transition from the school setting into the world of work is difficult for the majority of individuals. After periods of trial and error, changing jobs, and perhaps returning to school for additional training, a vocational adjustment is usually made. This is not to say that employment has been selected that will endure over the working lifespan of an individual, but employment stability has been realized and the movement to other employment can be accomplished with greater ease and confidence. For students who have a disability, this transition is often more difficult to achieve, takes longer and requires a variety of supportive services. These services can include, but are not limited to, counseling, vocational evaluation, work adjustment training, skill training, job placement assistance and job follow-up.

For those students who have suffered a severe brain injury, movement into competitive employment can present a unique challenge both to the student and to the vocational evaluator whose job it is to assist in determining an appropriate vocational goal. Problems other than vocational are also of paramount importance and must be addressed prior to and during the evaluation period. Concerns may include poor physical ability and endurance, limited cognitive abilities, inconsistent behaviors and lack of emotional control. It is important that the vocational evaluator rely upon other professionals to provide as much information as possible concerning the student so that all barriers to a successful vocational adjustment can be identified and addressed. Speech pathologists, physical therapists, occupational therapists, special education teachers, medical doctors, social workers, psychologists and rehabilitation counselors may provide information that is germane to the evaluator. Involvement of family members may also be a valuable resource in identifying strengths and potential problems. Once this information is collected and reviewed, a vocational evaluation plan can be formulated and implemented.

Developing Vocational Evaluation Strategies

As stated previously, each student with a brain injury is unique and the methods used by the evaluator must be comprehensive, addressing strengths and weaknesses. Perhaps the most effective evaluation tool is **situational assessment** which provides the evaluator with an opportunity to observe the student in a controlled work setting. Vocational evaluation units that are located within rehabilitation centers, schools, rehabilitation hospitals or universities offer excellent potential to develop situational assessment areas. Assessment sites are found within various work areas or departments in these locations and may include food service, mailroom, grounds maintenance, janitorial, switchboard/receptionist, shipping and receiving, and bench assembly. The cooperation of each department head and employees within each department is essential if this phase of the evaluation is to be a viable tool. It is the responsibility of the vocational evaluator to provide personnel within the work areas with an understanding of why the student is there and their role during the assessment.

Feedback from the situational assessment can be especially valuable in determining employment potential. Observations that are important can include productivity, endurance levels, punctuality, co-worker interaction, attentiveness to task and motivation toward entering competitive employment.

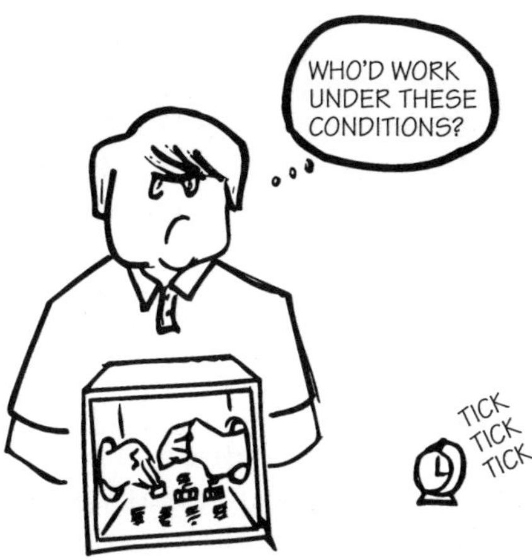

Standardized testing, including work samples and psychometric testing, is also a valuable tool to the vocational evaluator and is used to measure the following:

1. Motor Coordination
2. Finger and Manual Dexterities
3. Vocational Interests
4. Aptitudes
5. Academic Achievement Levels
6. Intellectual Levels

The evaluation report should not only discuss the test results, but should also reflect the problems that were identified during the evaluation and how they can best be resolved. In many instances, movement into a sheltered workshop, work hardening program or a supported employment program is initially a more realistic option than direct job placement. It is important that the student's progress in any of the above programs is monitored by a vocational counselor or case manager and that problems that present barriers to competitive employment are addressed. The primary goal, of course, is to provide the students with an opportunity to sustain themselves in a competitive work situation and to provide them with the skills to function independently both on and off the job. In order to successfully integrate students with brain injury into competitive work situations, both employers and workers must understand their roles. Employers must be aware of the unique needs of new employees, understand that they may experience difficulty in adjusting to the work setting, and be aware that physical, cognitive and behavioral problems can interfere with productivity.

Supported Employment

Another technique to ease the transition into competitive employment is supported employment which incorporates the services of a job coach. The responsibility of the job coach is to assist with job placement and provide on-going follow-up. The job coach can use the vocational evaluation report to identify potential areas of employment and vocational strengths and weaknesses. Roles of the job coach would include the following:

1. Educate the employer in the student's vocational strengths and potential areas of difficulty.

2. Train the student/employee in job duties.

3. Facilitate communication between the student, employer and co-workers.

4. Identify the need for job modification, including assistive devices, as well as techniques in performing the job duties.

5. Conduct follow-up in order to address potential areas of difficulty.

NOW WE'RE GOING TO
GO IN THERE AND PUNCH
THE TIME CLOCK.

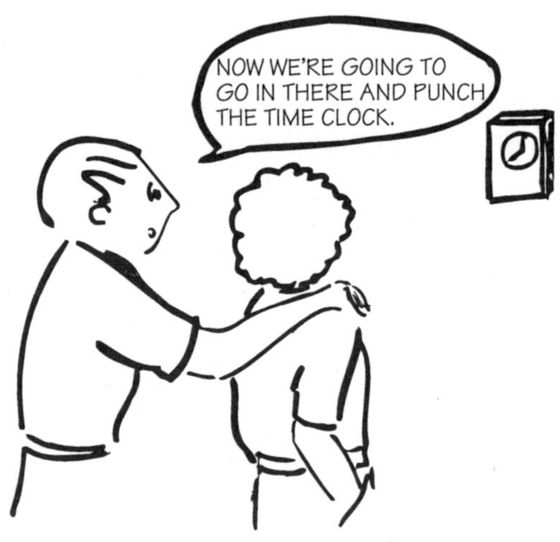

Important also to note is the quality of communication between the job coach and employer. Too often, small problems at the worksite are not brought to the job coach's attention or are trivialized by the supervisor. The problems have "snowballed" into a vocational issue in which employment may be jeopardized. Educating the supervisor will assist the student in becoming a more effective worker. Another important point is that simple job modification can be introduced to overcome physical obstacles such as those resulting from hemiparesis. For example, handles can be attached to a mop or broom to provide leverage, and knives with a special guard are available for safety purposes. Job coaches also work in cooperation with the student's family, if possible, to develop support at home. Supported employment which includes the involvement of a job coach goes beyond traditional job placement techniques. The goal of supported employment is to keep the student competitively employed by heading off potential job ending difficulties.

An example of a situation which would have possibly benefited from a job coach occurred when a head injured client was placed with a public utility company as a kitchen helper in the cafeteria.

Considerable time was spent with the food service staff and supervisor to orient them to the needs of this individual, and in acclimating the new employee to the responsibilities of the position. He was successfully employed for over three years without encountering any major difficulties. Unfortunately, the supervisor retired and a less understanding replacement was hired. The client became increasingly frustrated with the different approach used by the new supervisor, job performance subsequently deteriorated, and the client was let go after less than three weeks. It is important that employers are aware of possible problems and are provided with knowledge that will enable them and their staff to deal with difficulties as they arise. Supported employment can be an important consideration if the student requires on-going, long-term services in order to become and remain competitively employed. With supported employment, employers will have available the services of a job coach when needed and, in some cases, services can be provided indefinitely. In the case cited, supported employment was in place for the first six months of the student's employment. Had this time period been extended or had the new supervisor been aware of this service, perhaps the outcome would have been different.

Funding Sources

When services are not covered by insurance, the state office of vocational rehabilitation can provide funding for vocational services such as work adjustment training, vocational evaluation, skill training, job placement, supported employment and rehabilitation engineering. The student would need to make application for services directly with the state office of vocational rehabilitation.

Conclusion

Because of the multitude of deficits the student with brain injury may face, the evaluator often finds the standard vocational evaluation extremely difficult to implement. The majority of vocational evaluators do not generally receive specific training that enables them to perform evaluations with students with brain injury. In addition, most evaluation units do not receive a significant number of referrals involving this disability and evaluation expertise has been slow to develop. The evaluation can, however, incorporate techniques that have been proven useful in working with individuals with brain injury. These can include the following: frequent personal attention, speaking in short, clear sentences, providing frequent breaks, testing on a half day basis, allowing the evaluee to write out instructions, asking the evaluee to repeat instructions to insure that instructions are understood, and avoiding timed tests when possible. It is also important to provide praise and to use tests which will result in some success to the student. Also, the evaluator can help students realize that they are an important part of the evaluation process by explaining why tests are being administered and why it is important to put forth a positive effort on all assignments. Lastly, and foremost, students with brain injury must be treated with respect and understanding, and learn that their success is also the success of those individuals who have undertaken the responsibility of working with this most difficult population.

XI. SUMMARY

This book is being presented at a time when significant changes are occurring in the education of students with brain injury. The success of educating children with a brain injury is largely dependent on family members and educators 1) understanding both the dynamics of brain injury and the complexity of the interaction of students' capacities, skills, behaviors and environment, and 2) implementing effective strategies for intervention.

Recent advances have enabled us to improve our diagnostic and assessment capabilities so that children misdiagnosed or inappropriately diagnosed are correctly identified. Legislation at the federal and state level is beginning to yield recognition of brain injury as a separate disability category, making appropriate treatment programs possible. Other legislation is beginning to make funding available for remediation programs.

It remains for us as family members and professionals who will impact these young lives, to bridge a final gap — to actually incorporate and implement pertinent and appropriate strategies, with respect and understanding, knowing that as we provide quality educational (and vocational) services to our young people, we are not barriers to their success, but instead are enabling them to successfully meet the challenges in their lives.

XII. BIBLIOGRAPHY

Adamovich, Brenda B., Jenifer Henderson, and Sanford Auerbach. Cognitive Rehabilitation of Closed Head Injured Patients: A Dynamic Approach. College Hill Press, San Diego, California, 1985.

Cruickshank, William M. Learning Disabilities in Home, School and Community. Syracuse University Press, Syracuse, New York, 1977.

Cruickshank, William M., Frances A. Bentzen, Frederick H. Ratzburg, and Miriam T. Pannhauser. A Teaching Method for Brain-injured and Hyperactive Children. Syracuse University Press, Syracuse, New York, 1961.

DeBoskey, D. An Investigation of the Remediation of Learning Disabilities Based on Brain-Related Tasks as Measured by the Halstead-Reitan Neuropsychological Test Battery. Unpublished Doctoral Dissertation, University of Tennessee, 1982.

DeBoskey, D. Coming Home: A Discharge Manual for Families of the Head Injured. HDI Publishers, Houston, Texas, 1995.

DeBoskey, D., C. Calub, J. Burton, and K. Morin. Life After Head Injury: Who Am I? HDI Publishers, Houston, Texas, 2nd Edition, 1995.

DeBoskey, D., C. Dunse, J. Burton, L. Lowe, C. Cook, and D. McHenry. Teaching the Head Injured: What to Expect. HDI Publishers, Houston, Texas, 2nd Edition, 1995.

DeBoskey, D., C. Dunse, and K. Morin. Educating the Mild to Moderately Head Injured Child: A Neuropsychology Based Program. Tampa General Hospital, Tampa, Floida, 1986.

Dunn, Lloyd M. Exceptional Children in the Schools. Editor, Holt, Rhinehart and Winston, Inc., New York, New York, 1963.

Erikson, M.T. Child Psychopathy, Assessment, Etiology, and Treatment, pp. 204-251. Prentice-Hall, Inc., Englewood Cliffs, New Jersey, 1978.

Ewing-Cobbs, L., J.M. Fletcher, and H.S. Levin. Neuro-behavioral Sequelae Following Head Injury in Children. Journal of Head Trauma Rehabilitation, 1(4), 57-65, 1986.

Gearheart, B.R. and M.W. Weisbahn. The Handicapped Child in the Regular Classroom. The C.V. Mosby Company, St. Louis, Missouri, 1976.

Ginsburg, Herbert. Children's Arithmetic: The Learning Process. D. Van Nostrand Company, New York, New York, 1977.

Goldstein, Michael and Sam Goldstein. A Parent's Guide to Attention Deficit Disorders in Children. The Neurology, Learning & Behavior Center, Salt Lake City, Utah, 1986.

Howell, Kenneth W., Joseph S. Kaplan, Christine Y. O'Connell. Evaluating Exceptional Children, A Task Analysis Approach. Charles E. Merrill Publishing, Columbus, Ohio, 1979.

Kaufman, A.S. and N.L. Kaufman. Kaufman Assessment Battery for Children. American Guidance Service, Circle Pines, Minnesota, 1983.

Kaufman, James M. and Daniel P. Hallahan. Teaching Children With Learning Disabilities. Charles E. Merrill Publishing, Columbus, Ohio, 1976.

Keat, D.B. Multimodal Therapy With Children. Pergamon Press, Inc., New York, New York, 1979.

Kephart, Newell C. The Slow Learner in the Classroom. Charles E. Merrill Publishing, Columbus, Ohio, 1960.

Levin, H.S. and N.M. Eisenberg. Neuropsychological Impairment After Closed Head Injury in Children and Adolescents. Journal of Pediatric Psychology, 4, 389-402, 1979.

Mallison, R. Education As Therapy. Special Child Publications, Seattle, Washington, 1968.

National Head Injury Foundation. What Educators Need to Know About Students With Traumatic Brain Injury. The National Head Injury Foundation, Inc., Framingham, Massachusetts, 1985.

Peters, Ruth A. Who's In Charge. Lindsay Press, Inc., Clearwater, Florida, 1990.

Reitan, R. M. and D. Wolfson. Neuroanatomy and Neuropathology. Neuropsychology Press, Tucson, Arizona, 1985.

Reitan, R. M. and D. Wolfson. Traumatic Brain Injury -Volume I Pathophysiology and Neuropsychological Evaluation. Neuropsychology Press, Tucson, Arizona, 1986.

Savage, Ronald C. and Gary F. Wolcott. Educational Dimensions of Acquired Brain Injury. PRO-Ed, Austin, Texas, 1994.

Strauss, Alfred A. and Laura E. Lehtinen. Psychopathology and Education of the Brain-Injured Child. Grune and Stratton, Inc., New York, New York, 1947.

Wolcott, Gary F., Marilyn Lash and Sue Pearson, Signs and Strategies for Educating Students with Brain Injuries: A Practical Guide for Teachers and Schools. HDI Publishers, Houston, Texas, 1995.

Wood, R. L. Brain Injury Rehabilitation: A Neurobehavioral Approach. Aspen Publishing, Rockville, Maryland, 1987.

Ylvisaker, Mark. Children and Adolescents' Education. College Hill Press, San Diego, California, 1985.

Ylvisaker, Mark. Head Injury Rehabilitation: Head Injury Rehab With Children and Adolescents. Volume 12 in the HDI Professional Series. HDI Publishers, Houston, Texas, 2nd Edition, 1996.